Ron Gilbert
Kenneth W. Thomas · Gerd Schaller

SIDE EFFECTS

The Hidden Agenda of the Pharmaceutical Drug Cartel

Side Effects, The Hidden Agenda of the Pharmaceutical Drug Cartel
by Ron Gilbert, Kenneth W. Thomas, and Gerd Schaller.

ISBN 978-0-9819101-0-9

Editor: Linda Asato,
Present Time Books
500 N Osceola Ave. #411, Clearwater, Florida 33755 USA
Ph. 727-466-9772
Email: presenttimebooks@yahoo.com
Website: www.presenttimebooks.com

CONTENTS

WHAT IS A "DRUG"?

"1. Medicine, esp. a pharmaceutical preparation,
2. A substance taken for its narcotic or stimulant effect, often illegally."

(THE NEW OXFORD AMERICAN DICTIONARY)

First and foremost, the term *drug* points to a pharmaceutical, medical preparation. The word stems from the French word "drogue," meaning "chemical material."

Narcotics and stimulants include caffeine (in coffee), tobacco, alcohol, marijuana (colloquial: grass, pot, Mary Jane, cannabis, etc), heroin, cocaine, LSD, peyote/mescaline, and many other plant or animal-products, including pharmaceutical stimulants and the modern designer drugs.

In this book, when the word *drug* is used, it is usually with the meaning of the first definition, indicating the pharmaceutical preparation.

It seems to be more than revealing that the term *drug*, pointing to those highly dangerous, narcotic/stimulant substances leading usually to addiction, hallucination, sickness, pain and death (definition 2), is the *same* term, which we use today for pharmaceutical preparations (definition 1).

1. THE FUTURE OF A DRUGGED SOCIETY

We are all praying to a new God these days, and this deity is called "drug." Thus, we are made into believers of a new religion – the drug religion. How does a society get to a point where it believes that a drug is an answer to life's problems? With drugs, we believe we can solve all difficulties. Well, we soon discover that it doesn't solve them. When we get sick, we think a drug will help to make everything fine again. We come to believe, by the bombardment of suggestive advertising on TV and radio, and in magazines and newspapers – sometimes subtly and sometimes with force – that a drug will take care of our emotional duress. When we have disagreements with our partners, there is a drug that will fix that, too.

So "sayeth" the drug pushers, the pharmaceutical industries, and the companies that earn billions of dollars from their drugs every year. This unreflecting belief in drugs is nothing less than an intellectual scandal. The covert and overt efforts in making people believe that a drug is always the savior covers the fact that this society is heading in a totally wrong direction.

What are drugs really doing? What are the true side effects of drugs? What are their effects on a short-term and a long-term basis? Here are some of the effects of a society praying to drugs, according to critics, which we will quote later:

LESS SELF-RESPONSIBILITY

It's a stupid and incorrect credo that says, "With a pill everything can be solved." Of course, we are not speaking about someone who has to take heart medication in order to save his life as in the worst-case scenario. There are definite exceptions where medication is the right solution.

LESS RESPONSIBILITY FOR OTHERS

A drug, a pill, a doctor will take care of the problem of our fellow man, not you, the drug priests say. "You are not responsible for your feelings or actions."

NEW DISEASES

Some medications can create even more diseases, which will, in turn, be fought against by what? Yes, drugs of course. This is a downward spiral, and more and more drugs are the end result. So, at the moment we move in the direction of a DRUG SOCIETY.

LESS WORK, MORE SUICIDE

Psychoactive drugs can create more mental problems and can turn people into zombies making them less able to work. In the worst-case scenario, psychoactive drugs can lead to SUICIDE.

HIGHER WELFARE COSTS

Hospitals, doctors, etc, can be more expensive and the insurance costs may continually increase.

AN ENDANGERED OLDER POPULATION

The older population is especially overloaded with drugs today. The side effects are alarming, shortening the life spans of many.

ENDANGERED CHILDREN

Children who take psychoactive drugs are known to be less able to be educated, have a higher dropout rate, and have been shown to have a higher suicide and homicide rate. When we engage in a wholesale drugging of our children, it may very well be that we lose our future.

The pharmaceutical industries will be the obvious, big winner. They are already the number one moneymakers on this planet. They will use that Money Empire and lobby to gain control over governments, sports, anti-aging movements, older people, young people, and many social activities. *Capital control* by the big pharmaceutical companies will be the case.

One could break this problem down into a three-stage perspective:

Stage one is yesterday. The development of the first pharmaceutical drugs took place. Some demonstrated to be useful, to a degree, if not applied too long and not overused.

Stage two is today. The overuse of drugs for everything that ails us has occurred and we have the formation of a new drug religion. The "drugs can solve everything" attitude is spreading. Not being confronted are the incredulous side effects. Society is heading towards a dark future.

Stage three: if this trend continues, we will face a society even more controlled by the big drug companies (the legal drug pushers) and a Drug Society in a few tens of years.

So far, we've given you the bad news. Now, it may seem that this is a little bit of a black picture, too pessimistic, and not true. But don't forget to what degree we are already the effect of excessive advertisement, faking a wonderful new world with drugs.

The first indicators of a weak, irresponsible society brought on by drugs according to some critics (which are quoted later in this book) – with more crime, less literacy, and more stupidity – are already present. Covertly and overtly, the mighty pharmaceutical industry suggests another picture.

Perhaps drugs and medication are among the most important problems that we face today. Here we have problems that have dimensions no one dares to talk about or look at, because the consequences are too horrifying. The health care system will explode, willy-nilly, which will then, in turn, create higher taxes. This will lead to a lowered economic standard, and more poverty will ensue. Here we have a chain reaction.

But the financial and economic side effects are really only one side of the coin. The real side effects that are barely being confronted by anyone are the mental effects. One should never ignore the long-term side effects of drugs. Some have never truly been scientifically established. From various quarters, we hear about these horrible side effects. For example, mercury (which has been used in many vaccinations)[1] is said to have caused many new diseases and disorders. But this is only the tip of the iceberg.

1 In 2007, the manufacturers of vaccine have leaned more away from the use of mercury in their products.

According to the government's General Accounting Office (GAO), more than half of the prescription drugs (between 1976 and 1985) caused serious side effects.

Many resulted in hospitalizations, permanent disability and death.[2]

According to Public Citizen Research Group (PCRG), 119 out of 365 most commonly prescribed drugs for older people should not be used.[3] Sixty-one thousand people came down with Parkinson's disease.[4] There are 29 drugs on the market that can cause Parkinson's.

In addition to this:

65 can cause dementia
86 can cause depression
105 causes hallucinations
46 can make you fall and break bones
22 can cause auto accidents
119 causes sexual problems
88 causes constipation
18 keeps one from sleeping well.

(Source PCRG)[5]

According to a report of the American Medical Association (AMA), more that 100,000 Americans die every year from prescription drugs and over-the-counter medicines; 21,000,000 are seriously injured. Currently, drug reactions are the world's fourth major killer.[6]

The true side effects of the overuse of drugs lead to a DRUG PERSONALITY. A person dependent on medication is not unlike someone who is dependent on street drugs like marijuana…etc.

2 USA General Accounting Office. Report to the Chairman, Subcommittee on Human Resources and Intergovernmental Relations, Committee on Government Operations, House of Representatives: FDA Drug Review Postapproval Risks 1976-85. Washington, DC: USA General Accounting Office; 1990:3.

3 http://www.brwwellness.com/three.htm

4 Parkinson's disease: a brain disease that causes tremor and makes muscles rigid

5 Quoted from http://www.brwwellness.com/three.htm

6 http://www.yourhealthbase.com/database/a78d.htm

What are some of the manifestations of a DRUG PERSONALITY? From direct observation, one can see a person who is emotionally blunted. When a life situation calls for a normal emotional response for that situation, these people act woodenly – "zombie-like" – and inappropriately. For instance, if someone is given bad news such as the death of someone close, this person may not cry or experience grief as one would normally. If such a person sees an atrocity happening in front of them, as in the case of a criminal stealing an elderly lady's purse, they would not react or even become angry and try to stop the criminal. They might not even help the elderly lady after the perpetrator leaves the scene, leaving her distraught and fending for herself. Drug personalities operate their life around their medications. Without being medicated first, they won't do anything. If you want to do something spontaneous and they are not prepared for it, like a sudden trip to the shopping mall, these people would have to prop themselves up with medication to be able to confront the people and actions of going to the mall. They know when their drugs are effective or not and plan their lives accordingly. Being around a drug personality is like living with an alcoholic in that they don't do anything without access to their drug. Hiding and stealing, they make decisions that are detrimental to their families and friends, and act just like any other addictive personality. They believe that the drug makes them normal while actually it is quite the contrary.

One may say that this sounds all very well, but where is the proof for all these statements and for this bleak vision? More importantly, where are the alternatives?

Well, that's a good question!

Those statements have to be proven. We must have the exact data, numbers, tests, and scientific findings. This, we will do in the following chapters.

Let us start with the most controversial topic: MONEY. The most fearsome fact is the fact that the pharmaceutical companies already own an overwhelming amount of money.

But how much?

2. THE PHARMACEUTICAL INDUSTRY AND BIG MONEY

To say the pharmaceutical industry is a big moneymaker is an understatement. In fact, it is THE big moneymaker today. "Since the 1980s, the pharmaceutical industry has consistently ranked as the most profitable industry in the United States – by a long shot."[7]

Critics called the pharmaceutical industry "the other drug cartel" (*Office of the Minnesota Attorney General*), and pointed to their unbelievable profits, their political activities of the pharmaceutical industry, and their questionable lobbyism. In fact "... combined profits for the ten drug companies in the Fortune 500 ($35.9 billion) were more than the profits for all the other 490 businesses put together ($33.7 billion)."[8]

To really understand the pharmaceutical industry, one should just take a look inside the business. So, let us pick out just one example: *ASPIRIN*. Aspirin is the best-sold drug of all times. In the USA alone, 10,000 tons (yes, TONS) are sold every year.[9]

How did this story start?

AN UNBELIEVABLE SUCCESS STORY

Aspirin, the best-selling drug of all times, got its start in 1500 BC. The Chemical Heritage displays hieroglyphs depicting plants that the Egyptians used such as myrtle. Myrtle contains *salicylic acid* (SAS), a chemical compound we don't have to understand; we only have to know that this is the most important compound

7 Center for Policy Alternatives, "Playing Fair: State Action to Lower Prescription Prices," 2000

8 Public Citizen Congress Watch, "2002 Drug Industry Profits: Hefty Pharmaceutical Company Margins Dwarf Other Industries," June 2003 (www.citizen.org/documents/Pharma_Report.pdf). The data are drawn mainly from the Fortune 500 lists in *Fortune,* April 7, 2003, and April 5, 2004, and drug company annual reports.

9 See Kurt Langbein, Bert Ehgartner, *Das Medizin Kartell*, (München: Piper, 2002)

present in aspirin – it is the *secret* of aspirin if you wish. So, in the beginning, there was nothing more than a plant, myrtle. But the recorded dates vary. Others think that the birth of *aspirin* was somewhere between 460 BC – 377 BC, when Hippocrates, the famous Greek doctor, prescribed chewing on the bark of the willow tree to reduce fever and pain. The bark and leaves of the willow tree are rich in a substance called *salicin.*

Even the ancient Romans recorded the use of willow bark as a fever-fighter. In addition, there were many others over the years who found that making an infusion using birch bark and willow bark resulted in a useful pain reliever.

And then the age of chemistry began.

A French chemist named Charles Frederic Gerhardt was the first to synthesize *acetylsalicylic acid.* However, he failed to understand the properties and thus did not have any useful marketable material. He failed to become a billionaire, in other words. It took quite a few other investigators to create the wonder-pill, aspirin. These were the steps:

* In 1826, two Italians found that the willow bark's active ingredient was *salicin.*
* The Swiss pharmacist, Johann S. F. Pagenstecher, worked on the subject.
* German chemist, Karl Jacob Löwig (1803-1890),[10] experimented further.
* In 1859, Herman Kolbe synthesized *salicylic acid* using a coal tar formula.
* In 1869, Karl-Johann Kraut became the first scientist noted to accurately pin down the molecular structure of *salicylic acid.*
* In 1874, *salicylic acid*, using Kolbe's method, was sold as a painkiller in Dresden, Germany. But alas, this compound severely irritated the stomach.

10 Roy Porter, *The Greatest Benefits to Mankind,* (New York: W. W. Norton & Company, 1998)

And now begins the real success story.

In 1897, a chemist named Felix Hoffmann worked for the German pharmaceutical giant, *Bayer.* He was driven by the desire to find a cure for his father's arthritis, and decided to give Gerhardt's work another chance. The result was a huge success, and *Bayer* labeled it "aspirin."

The name, aspirin, was derived by using the "a" from *acetyle chloride*, the "spir" from the biological name of the plant (*Spirae ulmaria)* and the *in*, because it was the widely used ending for medication during that time.[11]

Imagine the excitement that Hoffman felt. One has to understand, somewhat, the emotion when aspirin became popular. Suddenly, or so it seemed, *pain* could be defeated. Doctors, patients, and chemists were overjoyed. And of course, so was *Bayer*, the pharmaceutical giant. Money, money, money flooded into the pockets of the pharmaceutical giant.

Please note that the founding father of the *Bayer group* was Friedrich Bayer, born 1828. He was nothing more than a dye trader, a son of a silk worker. He made money by establishing a huge, distribution network, reaching from London to Brussels, from St. Petersburg to New York. Finally, he used the discoveries of inorganic chemistry in the field of dyestuff. Later, *Bayer* expanded into the field of pharmaceuticals with the "drug of the century."

Aspirin was launched into the market in 1899. Quickly, the pharmaceutical department and an international presence were established. Nearly every country became involved and aspirin was suddenly the talk of the day. Already by 1913, approximately 10,000 people were employed by *Bayer*. Talk about success!

In the beginning, *Bayer* distributed aspirin powder to physicians only. Later, it became available without a prescription and was manufactured in tablet form. In 1920, it was even used to treat symptoms of pain related to rheumatism, lumbago, and neuralgia.[12]

---

11 http://www.chemheritage.org/EducationalServices/pharm/asp/asp180.htm

12 See Bayer AG-Company history 1881–1914. Print view http://www.bayeraspirin.com/pain/asp_history.htm

"An aspirin a day," was said, "could reduce even the risk of heart attack." And here we should wake up.

Heart problems – that was really something.

People died often – too often – because of heart attacks. It wasn't long before, aspirin was marketed as a pill against heart attack. A new market was born, new dollars; new billions of dollars were made. PR-geniuses even managed to get *Bayer* aspirin tablets included in the self-medication kits taken to the moon by the Apollo astronauts. But more importantly, a former, pain relief pill was instantly a potential lifesaver. Strokes, infarction[13] – suddenly a pill existed to prevent it. What a gigantic business! *Bayer* flourished and prospered.

Bayer (who also produced war material, including explosives, and chemical weapons) survived World War I and also World War II.

In 1925, Bayer transferred its assets to I. G. Farbenindstrie AG; although, we won't go into the war crimes of I. G. Farben, like providing killing gases for the concentration camps. For our purposes, it is only important to know that one day the sun shone again on *Bayer*. The worldwide connections were reestablished; *Bayer* joined with *Deutsche BP* to found *Erdölchemie GmbH*, successfully entering the petrochemical sector. But the pharmaceutical branch wasn't forgotten. Aspirin continued to be a huge success, again pouring billions and billions of dollars into *Bayer's* pocket. In 1963, *Bayer* employed nearly 80,000 people. Sales grew to approximately 4.7 billion DM[14] (1.2 billion USA dollars). Laboratories in the USA were bought. In 1987, 78% of the *Bayer Groups* sales were to customers outside of Germany.[15] In 1988, *Bayer* Sales amounted to 40 billion DM (10 billion dollars)! By that time, 165,000 people were working for *Bayer*. *Bayer* AG became the first German company on the Tokyo Stock Exchange. In North America, in Canada, in Japan, nearly everywhere, *Bayer* was

13 Infarction: an area of dead or dying tissue due to insufficient blood supply

14 DM: deutsche mark, German money

15 See http://www.bayeraspirin.com/pain/asp_history.htm

present. Think of the money *Bayer* made; think of the millions of dollars for the executives. As a note here, in 2004 Bayer reorganized into four operating subgroups, one of which is Lanxess, and three service companies under the umbrella of the management holding company. Lanxess took over the chemical activities and parts of the polymer business.

"A special highlight was the 100th birthday of aspirin in 1999, during which the company celebrated in spectacular fashion, transforming its high-rise headquarters building into a giant aspirin jack pack."[16] And this big THANK YOU had a reason. In 1998, the almighty Food and Drug Administration gave its sanction to new uses of aspirin. Aspirin now officially could be used to reduce the risk of death during a suspected heart attack, and prevent a recurrent stroke. In 2001, Bayer's shares started trading on the New York Stock Exchange; the Wall Street was enthused. During the *stock-market fever* time, *Bayer Group* reorganized, separations took place; new shares and new stocks were sold, and new names given. But *Bayer* (and its financial success) continued in 2005, 2006, 2007 and 2008. Today, Americans consume over 50 million aspirin tablets every day. That's over 15 billion tablets a year!

Judge for yourself. Aren't we living in a wonderful world? Isn't this super-success something we all should admire? And shouldn't we be happy that aspirin is with us, every day? Yes, we should be happy, if it weren't for those side effects. So let us look quickly at the other side of the coin.

SIDE EFFECTS

We constantly hear that "an aspirin a day will keep the doctor away." Is it an old wives tale or truth? Well, we know now that an aspirin a day has been recommended for people that suffer from heart attacks and strokes. We also heard that an aspirin could help in cases of aches and pains. What does this tiny little pill do that performs such miracles?

---

16 See http://www.bayeraspirin.com/pain/asp_history.htm

In a statement issued in January 2002 ("An Aspirin a Day – Good Medicine for Many," August 18 *Health Day News*), the *USA Preventive Services Task Force* concluded that there is excellent evidence that aspirin decreases the incidence of coronary heart disease in high-risk adults. Doctors, characteristically, suggest to patients with a history of heart disease and stroke to take the little magic pill to thin their blood. This would prevent the tiny blood clots from forming in certain conditions of diseases such as heart rhythms that go erratic, potentially leading to stroke, heart attacks often leading to death. According to the same article, "It's estimated that more than 26 million Americans are taking aspirin for their hearts."

Aspirin also helps with arthritis by reducing the inflammation of the joints where pain settles. And that's not all. Since aspirin aids with blood thinning for cardiovascular issues, it helps the blood flow easily through the veins and capillaries throughout the joint areas. Interestingly enough, doctors disagree about the exact dose of aspirin that patients should be taking. Many start their patients out at 81 milligrams, the equivalent of one baby aspirin or *low-dose* adult aspirin. Others recommend taking half of a standard 325-milligram aspirin daily, or one aspirin every other day. Logically, one may think that the lower the dose, the less the risk. But the only difference with lower dosages of aspirin is the longer amount of time that the side effects take to show up.

However, an aspirin a day could sometimes cause more harm than good, the *USA Food and Drug Administration* (FDA) warns. To take aspirin as a preventive measure can mean negative health consequences, such as stomach problems. But there are even more possible side effects such as:

- an allergic reaction (difficulty breathing; closing of your throat; swelling of your lips, tongue, or face, or hives);
- black, bloody, or tarry stools;
- nausea, vomiting, or abdominal pain;
- uncontrolled fever;
- blood in your urine or vomit;

- decreased hearing or ringing in the ears;
- seizures or dizziness, confusion, or hallucinations;
- heartburn or indigestion;
- faint ringing in the ears;
- drowsiness, or headache;
- excessive bruising resulting in hematomas (blood pooling under the skin into a clot).

On November 07, 2005, a message appeared in the news that aspirin diminishes the risk for skin cancer if you take this pill several times a day.[17] Why aren't the side effects published broadly as well?

Let's leave the subject at this point; in fact, we'll take the *true* story up again later. But at the moment, we don't want to destroy the joy you feel when you hear about the pharmaceutical industry's unbelievable success stories. So, let us quickly focus on another, more modern success-story.

VIAGRA

Let's change the medication and look at another modern, very exciting magic pill: *Viagra*.

Viagra is like champagne, in that it was discovered by accident. Dom Perignon set out to make a flat wine, but a secondary fermentation process put bubbles into it. Similarly, the pharmaceutical company *Pfizer* set out to make a drug that would relieve chest pain in patients with heart disease. An unexpected side effect was that the men in the test group who were receiving the drug began to have erections. So *Viagra*, starting its life as a pain reliever, became an aphrodisiac. We know that Dom Perignon was the inventor of champagne, but officially, at least, there is no one inventor of *Viagra*. The company line is that life might seem cruel, but the inventors are paid to work for the company, and the company owns their inventions. Literally hundreds of people at Pfizer have been involved in developing the drug. You can't

17 http://www.consumeraffairs.com/news04/2005/aspirin_skin_cancer.html

really point to two individuals and say they spawned *Viagra.* It is officially a drug invented by a cast of hundreds, perhaps thousands. A patent was granted for *Viagra* in 1996. The Federal Drug Administration (FDA) granted approval for the drug in March of 1998 and sales began shortly after that. It was the first drug approved for treatment of erectile dysfunction in the United States. Purchase of *Viagra* requires a prescription from a licensed physician. A marketing campaign for the pills included direct advertising to the consumers and included the endorsement of former senator and presidential candidate Bob Dole.[18] A blue pill in the shape of a diamond, Viagra (generic name Sildenafil) has become known as Vitamin V. The immediate success of Viagra was phenomenal since the incidence of "erectile dysfunction" was surprisingly high. Half of the men between ages 40 and 70 contract it at some point in their lives. After the age of 65, it's permanent in more than one out of every four men.

Viagra became an immediate success. Sales for the 1999 fiscal year topped one billion dollars and have been increasing ever since. By June of 1998, over one and a half million prescriptions were written. Then, by July of 1998, over three and a half million prescriptions were dispensed.[19] The huge revenue generated by *Sildenafil* sales has contributed greatly to the overall profitability of the drug company leading to an annual return for the pharmaceutical industry of 18.5%. This is quite high when one sees that the average Fortune 500 Company only returns 3.5% to its inventors. There has been a stable increase in drug revenues over time. From 1991 to 2001, drug revenues went from a 12.8% return to 18.5%. In comparison, the Fortune 500 return went only from 3.2% to 3.5%.[20] Even in 2003, when the profits of the other Fortune 500 industries were on a decline, big Pharma showed only a slight drop in profits (from 18.5% to 17% of sales).

18 Wikipedia, http://en.wikipedia.org/wiki/Viagra

19 Recreational Drug Information, http://www.a1b2c3.com/drugs/viagfaq.htm

20 Mike Hall, America at Work, http://www.aflcio.org/aboutaflcio/magazine/0503_bigfix.cfm

Before September 2004, there were no FDA-approved, generic substitutes for *Viagra*. *Pfizer* held a monopoly on this particular drug. But currently, there are two competitors, using a different technology. One of these, *Cialis*, has a 36-hour useful life rather than the few hours that Viagra has. It has already captured 18% of the Vitamin V market.[21] This and another competing drug were released in 2004, which have cut into Pfizer's market share by about 20%,[22] but there is still no reason for tears.

Pfizer owns multiple patents, which protect its proprietary interests in the drug. These patents are set to expire sometime between 2011 and 2013.

Of course there are a few side effects to the use of the drug. During testing of *Viagra*, patients reported problems with headache, rash, flushing of the skin, stomachaches, urinary tract infections, dizziness, diarrhea, and vision problems including blurriness and an inability to properly perceive light changes.[23] The vision problems restricted the user's ability to use heavy machinery and to drive a car.

An 18-page-long package insert accompanies the drug. It discusses the trials, but does not mention that anyone died during the trials, nor does it speak of any side effects. One interesting risk mentioned in the insert is that sexual activity is a risk factor for men with cardio-vascular health problems. Therefore, when a cardio-vascular case uses *Viagra* and engages in sex, he is more at risk for a heart attack. While the risk is not a direct side effect of taking the drug, the risk is directly connected to having sex while under the influence of the drug, the design purpose of the drug being to enhance the ability to have sex.

There are more side effects, but let us look at them later. For now, let's not be so negative and let's focus on success. To recapitulate, one pill alone made billions of dollars.

---

21 American Medical Network Cialis Could Top Viagra by 2006. September 2, 2004 http://www.health.am/ab/more1/cialis_could_top_viagra_sales_by_2006

22 Ibid.

23 Center for Drug Evaluation and Research, Federal Drug Administration http://www.fda.gov/cder/consumerinfo/viagra/viagrafaq.htm

Can you imagine anyone in the pharmaceutical company not liking *Viagra*?

OTHER GOLD MINES

To say that *aspirin* or *Viagra* are the only gold mines of the pharmaceutical industry would be far from the truth. To say that the pharmaceutical industry is continuously searching for new gold mines would be nearer to the truth. And yes, there are more and more incredible success stories.

Up to World War I, the pharmaceutical firm *Hoechst* (Germany) owned a monopoly on *Salvarsan*, which was supposed to heal syphilis. In the beginning, scientists warned about the horrible side effects (which included blindness, numbness, and paralysis, etc).[24] In addition to this, one out of every 200 patients died. But here was a market. So *Hoechst* worked like mad to develop a better product. Nevertheless, more than half of the 3,000 publications that appeared talked about the side effects.

Hoechst was even forced to publish all the possible side effects, which set the precedent so that today we have information in the form of a package-insert detailing possible side effects accompanying each pharmaceutical drug sold.

Despite all controversy, Salvarsan was a gold mine. But there were other gold mines. Each pharmaceutical company, today, has its gold mines. For example, in 2001, the number one pharmaceutical company, *Pfizer* (headquarters in New York, New York, USA) had as its top-selling products: *Lipitor*[25], *Norvasc*[26] and *Zoloft.*[27] Those three products brought the company $6.45 billion, $3.58 billion, and $2.34 billion respectively in one year alone. The company

24 See Langbein, p. 85

25 *Lipitor* is used to lower your *cholesterol. Cholesterol* is thought to be the cause of hardening the arteries and so a cause of heart-problems.

26 *Norvasc* is used to treat high blood pressure. It is also used to treat a type of chest pain called *angina*. Angina is often a pain or pressure in the chest that keeps coming back when part of the heart does not get enough blood.

27 *Zoloft* allegedly treats depression and panic.

GlaxoSmith Kline (headquarters in London, England) earned $2.68 billion with *Paxil*,[28] with *Augmentin*[29] $2.05 billion, and with *Flovent*[30] $1.32 billion.

Merck (headquarters in Whitehouse Station, New Jersey) won gold, silver and bronze in this Olympic race with *Zocor*,[31] *Vioxx*[32] and *Cozaar*,[33] ($6.6 billion, $2.5 billion and $1.9 billion).[34] We will recount the exact story of Vioxx later.

However, each of the giants in the pharmaceutical industry has top-selling products, and, in fact, one could go on and on, pages after pages, and quote those products, but the picture is always the same: the big pharmaceutical companies make their profit with just a few drugs.

So what does that mean? It simply means that the pharmaceutical industry is continuously looking for blockbusters, new magic bullets, and new and attractive markets. The money (and the survival) of the pharmaceutical companies depends to a great degree on some popular wonder-pills (drugs) which huge sectors of the population can use and are willing to do so.

If we could slip into the heads of the CEOs and marketing directors of those companies, we would see at a glance that those popular drugs, those best-selling pills, are the real goal.

So how does one create those bestsellers? By marketing research. One first defines a group of people, which one can *serve*. Then the job is to find their problems – the common denominator problems. After that one offers a solution to those problems, a new wonder-pill, and a magic bullet. And lastly one advertises like mad.

---

28 *Paxil* treats social anxiety disorder, depression and panic disorder.

29 *Augmentin* is an antibiotic in the class of drugs called penicillin.

30 *Flovent* aids in preventing asthma symptoms before they start.

31 *Zocor* blocks the production of cholesterol (a type of fat) in the body.

32 *Vioxx* is used to relieve the pain and inflammation caused by osteoarthritis. It is also used to relieve minor pain, headache, and menstrual pain and discomfort.

33 *Cozaar* is used to treat high blood pressure. It blocks the action of certain chemicals that tighten the blood vessels, so blood flows more smoothly.

34 See *Pharmaceutical Executive*, May 2002, pp 62, 63.

In theory, one can't even speak against this, because all companies want to survive; they want to make more and more money. This is the rule of the capitalistic world; this is the economic simplicity of it. And if those drugs did not have side effects, nobody could say anything against them. But here there is a big BUT. Before we come to that, let us take a look at the giants, the big players in the pharmaceutical industry.

TOP 10 PHARMA

Today, the pharmaceutical industry proudly presents its ranking.

The top ten are at the moment:[35]

1. Johnson & Johnson
2. Pfizer
3. GlaxoSmithKline
4. Novartis
5. Sanofi-Aventis
6. Hoffmann-La Roche
7. AstraZenca
8. Merck & Co
9. Abbott Laboratories
10. Wyeth

Five of them are located in the USA (*Pfizer*, *Merck*, *Johnson & Johnson*, *Abbott Laboratories*, and *Wyeth*), two in England (*GlaxoSmithKline* and *AstraZenca*), one in France (*Aventis*) and two in Switzerland (*Novartis and Hoffmann-La Roche*). The exact ranking varies from year to year.

Pfizer, the second biggest pharmaceutical giant, spends $17 billion every year for marketing alone and therefore belongs to the ten greatest advertisers in the USA.[36]

35 "Top 50 pharmaceutical companies," MedAdNews, September 2007

36 Der Spiegel 15/2005, p. 86

Germany, also, has a *great* tradition and history with the pharmaceutical industry. *Boehringer*, *Ingelheim*, *Bayer*, *Schering AG*, *Merck KGaA* and *Schwarz Pharma*, belong to the TOP 50 Pharma.

In Japan, the pill business is booming as well; about 10 of the top 50 today are Japanese firms. The pharmaceutical industry makes billions and billions of dollars every year. It is the biggest moneymaking machine in existence today on this planet. Especially, the top-selling products, which are important, bring in more than $1 billion each year. Unbelievable profits!

One doesn't need much imagination to see that the stockholders of pharmaceutical companies are very happy people. Their executives, especially when they buy stocks or stocks options, are even happier. Each of the top ten companies earns more than $11 billion on pills *alone*. Most products are sold in North America (about 55%), followed by Europe (about 20%) and Japan (about 18%). Even the Internet-fever Pharma is used for profit. Already top-selling products bought on line have their own ranking system. Some bestsellers on line include *Allegra* (treats seasonal allergies), *Effexor XR* (an antidepressant) and *Vioxx* (against arthritis pain). Again, we will cover Vioxx later.

And these are the real hard-hitting facts: "In 1999, the pharmaceutical industry has been the most profitable industry in the United States in each of the past ten years, approximately five and a half times more profitable than the average FORTUNE 500 company." (*Office of the Minnesota Attorney General*)

In 2002, health-care spending accounted for 15% of the USA economy. One doesn't need to be a prophet to see that, in 2006, 2007 and 2008, about 15% or more of the WHOLE USA ECONOMY would once again be built on health care. And here, blockbuster-pills are the most important subjects.

Money, money, money. An empire of money.

So the game is called *money*.

Allow me to make one more last remark. A car company can move its factories to Mexico and claim it's a free market. A toy company can outsource to a Chinese subcontractor and claim it's a free market. A major bank can incorporate in Bermuda to avoid taxes and claim it's a free market. We can buy HP printers made in Mexico. We can buy shirts made in Bangladesh. We can purchase almost anything we want from many different countries, BUT heaven help the elderly who dare to buy their prescription drugs from a Canadian or Mexican pharmacy. That's called un-American.

IT'S ALL ABOUT MONEY!

Did you ever wonder how much it costs a drug company for the active ingredient in prescription medications? Some people think it must cost a lot, since many drugs sell for more than $2.00 per tablet. We did a search of offshore chemical synthesizers that supply the active ingredients found in drugs approved by the FDA. A significant percentage of drugs sold in the United States contain active ingredients made in other countries. In our independent investigation of how much profit drug companies really make, we obtained the actual price of active ingredients used in some of the most popular drugs sold in America. The chart below speaks for itself:

DRUG NAME	100 TAB PRICE	ACTUAL COST	MARKUP
Celebrex 100 mg	$130.27	$0.60	21,712%
Claritin 10 mg	$215.17	$0.71	30,306%
Keflex 250 mg	$157.39	$1.88	8,372%
Lipitor 20 mg	$272.37	$5.80	4,696%
Norvasc 10 mg	$188.29	$0.14	34,493%
Paxil 20 mg	$220.27	$7.60	2,898%
Prevacid 30 mg	$44.77	$1.01	34,136%
Prilosec 20 mg	$360.97	$0.52	69,417%
Prozac 20 mg	$247.47	$0.11	224,973%
Tenormin 50 mg	$104.47	$0.13	80,362%
Vasotec 10 mg	$102.37	$020	51,185%
Xanax 1 mg	$136.79	$0.024	569,958%
Zestril 20 mg	$89.89	$3.20	2,809%
Zithromax 600 mg	$1,482.19	$18.78	7,892%
Zocor 40 mg	$350.27	$8.63	4,059%
Zoloft 50 mg	$206.87	$1.75	11,821%

Since the cost of prescription drugs is so outrageous, this helps to solve the mystery as to why they can afford to put a *pharmacy* on nearly every corner. Steve Wilson, an investigative reporter for Channel 7 News in Detroit, did a story on generic drug-price gouging by pharmacies. He found, in his investigation, that some of these generic drugs were marked up as much as 3000% or more. Yes, that's not a typo... 3000%! So often, we blame the drug companies for the high cost of drugs, and usually rightfully so. But in this case, the fault clearly lies with the pharmacies themselves. For example, if someone had to buy a prescription drug, and bought the name brand, he might pay $100 for 100 pills. The pharmacist might tell him that if he got the generic equivalent, they would only cost $80, making him think he was "saving" $20. What the pharmacist is not telling him is that those 100 generic pills may have cost the pharmacist only $10. So the pharmacies and the Big Pharma often work hand in glove. Both are responsible for rip-off prices.

So, it isn't very surprising that more pills are invented continuously. Especially, investments in Genentech and Biogen are the talk of the day.

Oil was once called black gold; pills are the new white gold. The best-selling product, *Zocor,*[37] was worth $6.6 billion in 2001. Approximately $300 billion are earned each year when it comes to pills. To summarize, altogether "the industry has been the most profitable industry in America for each of the past ten years." The years 2005, 2006 and 2007 didn't change that picture.

Who gets the advantages of that? Again in the first place, of course, it is the top-executives who get fantastic salaries, stock-options, bonuses, automobiles, travel-allowances and incentives. How much? A great deal! In Europe, in 2004, three out of eleven highest paid executives were pharmaceutical bosses. The magazine *DER SPIEGEL* estimated that *Novartis* paid his top-manager 12.75 million Euros (18.48 million dollars a year), *Aventis* paid 8.78

37 *Zocor* is used to reduce the total amounts of LDL (bad) cholesterol, triglycerides (another type of fat) and apolipoprotein B (a protein needed to make cholesterol) in the blood.

million Euros (11.6 million dollars), and *AstraZeneca* paid 4.47 million Euros (6.48 million dollars).

But there is more: *Families USA* researched the highest paid executives of nine pharmaceutical companies. "The average annual income, exclusive of unexercised stock options, was nearly $21 million in 2001."[38] The highest annual income was $74 million dollars. Per year!

Did those numbers change in 2008? We don't think so.

Good Lord! But aren't those salaries justified? Don't we live in a new world – a wonderful world of magic bullets that can solve everything, with which we allegedly can buy potency, sexual drive, longevity, health and even happiness? At least, this is what the new priests of the pharmaceutical companies tell us. One tends to believe that we are entering a new Golden Age, if – if – well, if there wouldn't be those side effects.

THE INVENTION OF NEW DISEASES

Before we come to those side effects, let us take a look at how new medications are created. One should not forget that each new wonder-pill, each new moneymaker means survival for a company. It means millions and sometimes, for its executives, a rich life and wealth. So *everything* is done to push new products. To detect a new gold mine (read new pill) that sells, one needs only to take certain steps. For the purpose of bringing a new blockbuster-pill to the market, one first has to define an exact public. So how is that done? It is done by definition of a new health-problem, for example. Or even better: by definition of a *risk factor*. Critics talk about the invention of new diseases.

Let's take a closer look at that. If one wants to define new *risk factors,* one just has to take a look at the statistics. What do the statistics say today? Well, in the USA, *heart disease* causes death in 31.4% of all cases, *cancer* in 23%, and *stroke* in 6%. You should also take a look (from the viewpoint of a pharmaceutical marketing

38 "Profiting from Pain," *Families USA*, p. 5

expert) at the facts of aging. PREVENTIVE MEDICINE and ANTI-AGING MEDICINE are popular today. Menopause and prostate problems are nearly inevitable when one enters a certain age.

Let's look at prostate problems. Three things can go wrong with the prostate gland: prostatitis (prostate infections), prostate enlargement (BPH) and prostate cancer. Now, instead of turning to better nutrition, natural treatments, engaging in more sports, cleansing the body from inside, and avoiding alcohol and drugs, one can look through the eyes of a pharmaceutical marketing expert. What will he see? A NEW MARKET. Since nearly every man, when he gets old enough, will develop prostate problems, one can invent a new product, which "one should take to avoid prostate problems before they arise."

Does that mean one shouldn't take precautions against prostate problems? No! Prostate problems *are* real, but there are lots of natural ways to deal with this problem. Does that mean that all prostate-problem pills are for the birds? No, not necessarily. It means that marketing experts are searching, looking continuously for new markets so that a blockbuster pill can be invented and sold. In the eyes of a marketing-expert, the following is true: the more people are potential buyers for a new magic bullet, the better. A pill that reaches ALL elderly people or a pill for ALL children – *that* is the real deal! When one can define risk factors for heart problems – wonderful. *What a market*! Why? People die in 31.4% of all heart-disease cases.

Let us look at one example. Uffe Ravnskov pointed out that "an expert panel" once defined new guidelines for "the detection, evaluation, and treatment of high blood cholesterol" (high blood cholesterol, some experts say, leads to heart-problems).[39] This "expert panel" published those new guidelines on May 16, 2001 in the Journal of the American Medical Association. New risk factors for heart problems were born; new demanding, preventive actions, according to this "expert panel," were necessary. The point is, once defined, new risk factors (like abdominal obesity, high blood

39 See Uffe Ravnskov, MD. PhD, independent research, Spo, http: www.opinions3.com/Uffe_Ravnskov_Report.htm

pressure, high fasting blood sugar) or a combination of several risk factors open up a new market. People with those risk factors, should do what? Yes, they SHOULD TAKE A SPECIAL PILL. Got it? Simple. Hurrah! A new market. New risk factors. A whole new target-group can be put on a pill. New billions in the pockets of the pharmaceutical industry. Is this new pill unnecessary? We're not even mentioning that. It's interesting that although 67% of the patients talk to their doctors about cholesterol, only 34% are advised to exercise and 37% are advised to quit smoking – obvious contributors to heart disease. Yes, many experts claim that many of those new "risk factor pills" are more dangerous than the possible disease, because of the side effects and because natural treatments are not done, but this is not even our point here.

Our point is the way those marketing gurus THINK. Critics (like Ray Moynihan, Iona Heath or David Henry – a professor of clinical pharmacology) call it "selling sickness" or "disease mongering." They talk about "widening the boundaries of treatable illness in order to expand markets for those who sell and deliver treatments."[40] They talk about the systematic medicalisation; they talk about turning "ordinary ailments into medical problems, seeing mild symptoms as serious, treating personal problems as medical."

There are complete sales strategies, which go along with this.

One strategy: involving the media, who like to create fear.

Another one: winning KOL (=key opinion leaders) and paying them a good salary so that those KOL give the necessary statements in public when needed.

Another one: financing tons of TV spots.

Another one: medically "educating" large groups of doctors in leading medical magazines.

Another one: sponsoring experiments with paid patients.

Another one: inviting doctors for "information holidays."

There are many ways to develop new markets. One can define a new phobia. (Not to say that there isn't a single human individual

40 http://bmj.com/cgi/content/full/324/7342/886

who lacks phobias.) Or one can take the older population and, instead of promoting Calcium and Magnesium for the old bones, develop a new wonder-pill. One can point to erection problems (as in the case of Viagra) and so on. FINDING new diseases. DEFINING new diseases. PROMOTING new diseases. That is the high-art of the pharmaceutical research expert. It is MARKETING KNOW HOW.

Did you ever notice the astonishing increase of new diseases today? Marshall Smith, editor from the BroJon Gazette, states in the article *Fever and the Mystery Disease Sars*,[41] "In the last 20 years, in my research, articles and media interviews, I have identified 12 fictitious medical problems, which have resulted in massive billion dollar profits to a few pharmaceutical houses. All of the medical problems were either man-made or don't exist, and were hyped and promoted by the CDC.[42] All of them are characterized by including the words Disorder or Syndrome in their names. That's because they are not legitimate diseases. I am sure we can think of a few of the big ones. I won't mention them here, since that would take us off the topic."

Allergies? Chronic Fatigue? Autoimmune problems? What a wonderful world where a new disease is found every day. The population gets hooked by its own fear. And so the pockets of the pharmaceutical industries are filled. Are we saying that every pill is nonsense and does not work? No.

We just mention HOW those marketing experts and PR geniuses think, compute, and operate. The economical pressure of continuous expansion dictates that behavior.

Listen to the radio yourself. See, with a critical attitude, the pharmaceutical advertisements on TV. Do you recognize how smart all this is? "If you have this and that, you MAY QUALIFY for this new pill…." The most genius minds, the highest paid marketing experts are hired by the pharmaceutical companies –

41 http://www.brojon.org/frontpage/SARSFEVER.html

42 CDC: Centers for Disease Control are different centers throughout the United States that are funded with private grant money from pharmaceutical companies to "discover fictitious disorders" and promote the pharmaceutical drugs.

they have the money to pay them. And so we are bombarded with risk factors.

The very competent authors, Langbein/Ehgartner, point out that millions of people can be recruited for a new medication just by defining a new risk factor. The cholesterol problem earns billion of dollars every year. The methodology is to talk about good and bad cholesterol and define new limits. Added hormones are another subject, altogether.

Oh! Hormones are becoming a household word. Suddenly, everybody talks about menopause, andropause, estrogen, testosterone, the female and the male hormones. Hormones are simply substances, formed in an organ of the body (gland), which is then carried to another organ (or tissue) where it fulfills a specific purpose. So, yes, hormones are important. But lately, some "experts" say that each person over 50, let us say, should check his or her hormones. Find out if your hormones are in balance. If not, do hormone therapy. "If your hormones are not in optimal balance you must act!" postulate the creators of the Hidden Agenda.

The actual truth of it is that there are so many natural means to balance out hormones, it is mind boggling. From nettle-root to Saw Palmetto, from Pygeum Africanum to vitamins.

But no, for sales purposes, a hormone-therapy is more rewarding.

Millions of healthy people can, by a new definition of risk factors, become patients – and a great source for the pharmaceutical industry income. High blood pressure? Low blood pressure? Fantastic! A new income source. That there are natural means to handle these is seldom mentioned. Why? No income for the industry.

People are too fat? Fantastic! A new income source. Fat people have a higher risk for this and for that. So you give pills, pills, pills. Instead of promoting a no-sugar diet, sports, less carbohydrates and more protein from natural sources that don't have hormones in them, you promote a pill. Blood sugar imbalanced? Oh, pure joy! Again a great market. More and more diseases are defined.

Bones a bit weaker? Great! A new star is borne. The star? A wonder pill.

Does that not make sense? Fantastic, fantastic new markets! New income sources! So what does that mean? Well, it simply means that, on the hidden agenda of the pharmaceutical drug cartel, there is *continuous* research for new risk factors. It is GOOD NEWS for the pharmaceutical drug industry when a new risk factor is found. That means a definition of a new target group. With every new "finding," with every new risk factor, with every new definition of whatever biological parameter, new markets can be defined. Paradise! For the pharmaceutical drug cartel. Too much stress? Mmmm... let's look, perhaps we have a pill for that? Too old? Too fat? Still young and hyperactive? Bingo! Strengthening the heart means billions of dollars for the pharmaceutical industry. Smoking? Hmm... let's see if there is a market. Involved in sports? Hmm... let's see. Perhaps what is needed is *steroids*! See what I am getting at?

We are already living in a pharmaceutical-drug world. Very intensely, continuing new target markets are researched and defined. And the perspective is wonderful. Endless. The horizon is far away. No end, no limit for income. From the viewpoint of a pharmaceutical marketing-guru he could take old people, young people, sportive people, and risk-factors people. Good Lord! He could sell pills to nearly everybody in the end. So the hidden agenda of the pharmaceutical industry is just this: turn us into a drug-society. And nobody seems to know what the *real* side effects of a drug-society are. Taking a new pill is not a big deal anymore today. No big deal? Well, yes, if there wouldn't be those side effects.

But wait a minute! What about the unbelievable hurdles that exist for Big Pharma when they try to bring a new medication to the public? Bingo! Now it really becomes exciting. One may argue (and the pharmaceutical industry argues that way) that the development of new drugs is very expensive. And that LOTS of money has to be invested in R & D (Research & Development) of a new medication. Not true. Reports (e.g. from *Families USA*) reveal, "On average, companies spent 11% of the revenue on R & D and 27% of revenue on marketing, advertising and administration."[43] *Families USA* puts it this way: "It is clear that leading drug companies are marketing machines much more than they are pharmaceutical research houses."

Any more questions?

And it is true. Looking at the money, the Exec-Strata earns a lot. Looking at the sales efforts (hiring sales-representatives, marketing-gurus, PR-specialist, opinion leaders) – here is where the money is spent.[44] So let us quickly forget the fairy tale regarding the huge spending for R & D (for new medication). Yes, some is spent but not for the most part. Data shows big drug companies spent almost two and one half times as much on marketing, advertising, and administration as to research and development. Period. (Source: The book *Profiting from Pain* by Families USA) But there are even more hard hitting facts: "Experts estimate that up to 85% of R & D funding comes from National Institutes of Health (NIH), public tax credits, private foundations, and academia."[45] So even the "famous" research is not as famous as the pharmaceutical industries try to make us believe. *The Office of the Minnesota Attorney General* gives many examples for that. Here is just one: the breast cancer drug *Taxol*. This drug was develop by $32 million in federal funding and took 30 years of research. In 1992, the NIH licensed Taxol to Bristol-Myers Squibb, which then generated $2 billion of revenue *per year* on the sale of the product. So again, quite a few blockbuster medications are clearly developed by public funding, academic medical centers, and foreign academic centers, whilst the pharmaceutical industry gets additional tax-advantages. So, in what are the pharmaceutical companies investing? Yes, in advertising, advertising, advertising. And in sales, sales, sales. The physicians are swamped with pharmaceutical sales representatives. And the physicians get "luxurious information" about the merits of a new

43 *Families USA,* Pp. 5,10

44 "Profiting from Pain where Prescription Drug Dollars Go," report by *Families USA*, July 2202, Washington

45 Follow the Money, The Pharmaceutical Industry – the other Drug Cartel, Office of the Minnesota Attorney general, Sept 30, 2003 p. 1

product, sometimes in a great environment of course. Here billions of dollars are spent every year. Listen to the radio; watch the TV with open eyes. What do you hear and see?

How does Big Pharma manage to come away with that?

LOBBYISM AT ITS BEST

We don't want to talk about the critics who point out that the "unbelievably careful studies" which are done with each new medication are not "unbelievably careful." We also don't want to talk about the fact, that Peter C. Gotsche, director of the Nordic *Cochrane-Center* in Copenhagen, checked all major studies about mammography-inquiries (for detecting breast cancer); six out of eight inquiries had major methodological mistakes, some were on the borderline to manipulation.[46] Authors of the British magazine *New Scientist* stated that 80% of all medical actions that are taken don't meet high scientific standards. (Repeat: 80%.)[47]

We, also, don't want to point out the fact that independent researchers are, meanwhile, hard to find, meaning to say that most "clinical studies" are paid by the pharmaceutical industry. No wonder, where billions are pumped into the development of new medication!

We don't even want to mention that sometimes "scientists" are prevented from publishing results that are not needed and wanted by Big Pharma.[48]

We don't want to say, that 98% of all "scientists" who work for Pharma, give a positive judgment about a new medication. Without big money, only 79%[49] are positive.

We don't want to mention that Big Pharma is the closest friend of the physicians; that the doctors receive luxurious "information" in an awesome setting, and that Big Pharma spends LOTS of

46 Kurt Langbein p. 72

47 *New Scientist*, 17 Sept. 1994, p. 23 ff

48 Langbein, p. 339

49 (Cho, M.K., Bero, L.A. *The quality of Drug Studies, Published in Symposium Proceedings*, (Ann Intern Med 1996), 124 (5), Pp. 485-489

money to gain the support for new medications within the doctors' associations. Robert S. Mendelsohn stated, "Of course, in these instances, doctors working for drug companies have as their goal, producing results that will convince the FDA to approve the drug. Sometimes, with competition for grant money getting more and more fierce, doctors simply want to produce results that will keep the funding lines open. Since all the *good-ol'-boy* researches are in the same boat, there seems to be a great tolerance for sloppy experiments, non-confirmable results, and carelessness in interpreting results."[50]

In Germany, the health sector loses 20 billion euros (28.99 billion dollars) through corruption and betrayal, guesses *Transparency International*. One of the great spenders is the pharmaceutical industry! In United States, "scientific studies" are quite often falsified. The *Spiegel* reported, that every seventh researcher admitted to having falsified scientific studies, so that the end result pleases. Repeat: every seventh![51]

Here's how "scientific" research becomes falsified. Falsifications in so-called scientific communities have tradition. We know about Trofim Lysenko, who cheated the whole Russian scientific biology community. We know about William Summerlin, who falsified data in relation to skin transplantation. Cyril Burt lied about scientific result in his twin research. Ninety-four publications of Friedhelm Herrmann, a cancer researcher, were manipulated. And we have in recent times, of course, South Korean Hwang, once the superstar in relation to cloning human embryos, lying about new therapies – and the whole world believed it. Experts, like Andreas Diekman, state that falsifications and manipulations especially happen most often in the biomedical area; he says that side effects are sometimes just ignored; there are not enough systematic research done, or they are just plain manipulations.[52]

---

50 Robert S. Mendelsohn, *Confessions of a Medical Heretic*, (McGraw-Hill: 1980), p. 125

51 Der Spiegel 32/2005, p. 54

52 Der Spiegel, February, 2006, p. 156 f

We really don't want to say all that. Why? Because there is a much bigger scandal! There is even hotter information.

So what do we really want to say?

We want to speak about the *political* influence of the pharmaceutical industry. The purpose: to protect the profit. A survey, done by the *Attorney Generals Office Minnesota* (in which 17 pharmaceutical companies and their industry organization *PhRMA* were surveyed) demonstrated that the industry spent over $477 million lobbying the federal government in 2000-2001 alone. But that is nothing in relation to the following number. Drug companies today deploy an army of 675 lobbyists to protect their profits. Six hundred and seventy-five lobbyists exist – more than there are Senators and Representatives! These 675 people *continuously* try to influence politics. So what are they doing? They prowl the hallways of power in Washington to promote their drugs. In fact, this activity costs over $91 million.[53]

Dr. Ken Goldstein, Professor of Political Science University or Wisconsin, says (AARP Bulletin, Pulling Strings From Afar, February, 2003), "The drug industry is once again on track to be the biggest industry-group spender in American elections."[54]

Congressman Sherrod Brown puts it clearer. He stated that the pharmaceutical industry "is in the White House." Wall Street journalist, Tom Hamburger (Drug Industry moves to Bolster Image Before Vote, Sept 16, 2002), talks about contributions of millions and millions of dollars, which go to candidates and parties. And yes, groups that are accused of being financed by the pharmaceutical industry back candidates in favor of the pharmaceutical industry.

So an unbelievable amount of money flows to election campaigns.

In addition, lobby groups are put upfront, all with just one purpose: to influence politics. The trick is to *create* "front groups"

53 Marcia Angell, M.D., *The Truth about the Drug Companies*, (New York: Random House, 2004), p. 198

54 Pharmaceutical Companies http://ushealthcarereform.com/page8.html
Pulling Strings from Afar AARP Bulletin Today 2006-07-03 http://bulletin.aarp.org/yourworld/politics/articles/pulling_strings_from.html

with names that have a good PR value. Creating *misleading* names! And not disclose that Big Pharma finances those front groups. Especially under fire are those front groups, which have names to bring tears of joy to the eyes of every PR expert. "Citizens for a Better Medicare," "United Senior Associations," "Consumer Alliance" and others have been accused of being financed by the pharmaceutical industry, while giving the impression of being independent, a grass-root-organization. At the same time, lobbyists included 26 former members of Congress, and another 342, who had been on congressional staffs or otherwise connected with government officials. Some lobbyists, such as Scott Hatch, were actually related to members of Congress. Scott is the son of Senator Orrin Hatch. These relationships ensure that the pharmaceutical industry has the attention and sympathy of ears in Washington. Imagine that!

In the year 2000, President George W. Bush received $477,633.00, while senator Majority Leader Bill Frist (Republican TN) got $116,457.00 and Senator Orrin Hatch (Republican UT) $399,874.00, etc.[55] Politicians in favor of the pharmaceutical industry (i.e. voting for their interest) received more money than those voting against them, of course. Experts estimate that about two thirds of this money, which influence politicians, goes to the Republicans and one third to Democrats. In the 1999/2000-election cycle, the Republicans "received about 76% of the drug industry's financial largesse."[56] Lobbying Congress cost the pharmaceutical industry hundreds of millions of dollars. In the 2004 election year, with its surprising outcome, the mega-fundraisers of George W. Bush were also under attack. The Republicans differentiate between *Pioneers* (raising more than $100,000) and the *Rangers* (raising more than $200,000). Nothing wrong with this, despite critics have said that half of the Republicans funds come from those *Rangers* and *Pioneers,* and that this money doesn't represent "THE PEOPLE" anymore – but OK! What makes this money really interesting is

55 http://www.saynotodrugs.org/

56 John Abramson, M.D., *Overdosed America, the Broken Promise of American Medicine,* (HarperCollins Publishers, 2004,) p. 90

the fact that the Pharmaceutical Industry is one of the big spenders. *Bayer*, *PoxMeyer Heath Corp.*, *Maxor National Pharmacy*, *Direct Meds Inc, Pfizer*, and *AstraZeneca* all belong to the big spenders. Their executives or lobbyists funded Bush! So Big Pharma invests in lobbying, in front groups, in campaigns, in political parties. And the money, from the viewpoint of Big Pharma, is well invested. Authors of *Buying a Law* guess that a total of $671 million, over the period of some years, have so far been invested, and $139 billion (BILLION) were made in profits. A good deal! How was the money made? For example, by "buying a law" and insisting that USA citizens have to buy expensive drugs inside the USA and not cheaply from Canada. Not only that, the Third World Countries are prevented from producing or importing generic drugs in order to obtain medication for their HIV/AIDS victims. They are too poor to afford the high prices of medication from the United States. This opposition to relax the patent protection in a Third World country was carried out by both the Bush and Clinton administrations.

Author Peter Weaver concludes, "They [the pharmaceutical companies] use the power and the money to shape governmental policy, to support political candidates, and to manipulate public opinion in their favor. This relentless lobbying effort has one primary goal: to prevent any attempts by the USA government to control or limit the prices of prescription medicines."[57]

Change of subject: during the 2008 election cycle Democrats received about $4 million from the Pharmaceutical industry and the Republicans obtained close to the same amount. Is Big Pharma buying our politicians? Well the above numbers are facts, not a weird conspiracy theory.

Let us repeat: the industry is "spending" tons of money on the members of USA House of Representatives and the USA Senate. It goes to "decision-makers," to opinion leaders, to KOLs (Key opinion leaders). So what does that mean? Well it simply means that Big Pharma protects its profits.

57 Peter Weaver, *Smart Medicine, How to buy the prescription drugs you need a price you can afford*, (Nashville, TN: Rutledge Hill Press, 2004), p. 13

Look at the Drug Stores. Many are expanding nationwide. *Medicap Pharmacies, Walgreens, EVCs, Discount Drug Marts, Eckerds.* They look for expansion in the right place, the vicinity of supermarkets and aim at exact demographics, i.e. the middle-income people. In earlier times, the churches dominated the picture. Then the banks came and the insurance companies. Today the drugstores are everywhere. Money, money, money. We all know that the effort to make medications cheaper for the American citizens failed. The results? Today 23% of what Americans spend out of their pockets goes to health care (Health & Human, Services Department study, in Jan 2004). In other numbers, $155 trillion (Yes, Trillion!) were paid by people in the USA, or $5,440 by each individual person paid to *Big Pharma and Associates*.

These are simple facts.

A POSSIBLE SCENARIO

What does all this information tell us? And, more importantly, how will that change the future, when this trend continues? Well, hardly anyone *really* looks at the future of a society, which is dependent to such a degree on drugs – on medication! Let us give the scenario of when this TREND continues: Health Care controls 15% of every dollar in the USA today – 15%! Tomorrow it may be 20%, then 25%. It will increase. So we will have AN ECONOMY CONTROLLED BY THE PHARMACEUTICAL INDUSTRY! To a huge extent, at least. The spending of each and every single man and woman for pharmaceutical products will go up. Let us repeat: $155 trillion is already spent in America today for medical cost ($5,440 for every individual). Tomorrow, it will be *more*. Big Pharma will use the money to gain more and more *control*. We will have more super-rich people in the USA and in the industrialized world as well (in Germany, France, Japan, etc.) and a smaller middle-class will ensue. More people will move towards poverty. The middle-class will have more and more problems, just speaking strictly of finances. In many fields, Big Pharma will exert control, overtly and covertly.

The second effect will be in the political arena. Even today, it is already a scandal! The figures, speak for themselves. Again, we already have 675 Pharma lobbyists. Tomorrow, it may be 1000. The lobbyists will bombard the key opinion leaders. Big Pharma will decide if an election is won or not. Pharma will decide politics and influence law in the end. We will be manipulated into a pro-pharmaceutical world, where allegedly everything can be solved with drugs. Pharma will buy politicians, directly or indirectly, with more "front groups" with PR-strategies, marketing and sales efforts. The influences will have nothing to do with democracy in the end. Political "leaders" will be puppets on the strings of the pharmaceutical industry. In the long run, we will lose democracy, freedom of choice, power of choice. We will be controlled by a little circle of insiders who think in profits exclusively. Our hard-won, hard fought-for rights will be lost, not overtly in the beginning but covertly and we will end up with a tyranny dictated by a small group of people who can decide about our future.

The worst is not yet said. The true side effects, and by far the most dangerous ones, will be CONTROL OF THE MEDIA and thus CONTROL OF THINKING. Already today, people believe that drugs can fix everything; that drugs are the universal solver. Bombardment with seductive pictures is already a reality. Tomorrow, politicians can no longer say what they want. TV will be dependent on the purchase of advertisements by Big Pharma, and TV will suggest, hypnotize, and manipulate us into a blind belief in this new religion, this new God, called DRUG. Free thinking, free research, true science will be impeded along with the recognition that there are so many other ways to solve our problems. The overwhelming advertising, the billions of dollars spent here, will covertly and overtly corrupt the thinking of even the best of us. We will drop into a chemical, drug-oriented society.

Again: this is a *possible* scenario! You think that this is too black a picture? Well, we haven't even *begun* to tell the truth.

We haven't mentioned how bribery is committed, what the high art of corruption is, and which deceptive ways exist to deceive the public. We are just at the very beginning. And we haven't touched on the true side effects some drugs have on the body and the mind.

ULRICH SOMMER: "MANY OF THE MEDICATIONS JUST DO NOT WORK."

Before we go to the next chapter and between every chapter in this book, we have placed an interview with a professional so that the reader can have additional, first-hand information about the subject just talked about.

This has the advantage of giving the reader the opinion and evaluation of a top-expert in the field, unchanged through the author's viewpoint. You still get an authentic view by someone who was or is intimately connected to the scene or the topic.

The first interviewee is an expert when it comes to drugs insofar as he worked for a long time as a pharmacist in Germany. He studied the subject in Kiel, Germany, and took his state examination in 1971. He first worked as an employee in a pharmacy, from 1971 – 1973, and then, in 1974 – 1975, he ran his father's pharmacy with his brother. In 1975, he opened up his own pharmacy as a sole proprietor and ran it for about 14 years.

Ulrich Sommer has, therefore, a deep insight into the practices of the pharmaceutical industry, being part of the system himself for a long time. He had one of the best operating pharmacies in Germany. In 1989, he sold his pharmacy, realizing drugs often did more harm than benefit to the individuals he sold them to. He searched for products that created health instead of poor health and body conditions, and therefore founded a company based on these principals. Coming to the USA, he contacted researchers, scientists and explorers, who were very experienced in this field. In the following years, he built up an alternative sales/distribution business. His mail order company for herbs and nutritional supplements continued to expand and to this day he keeps looking for methods of how to stay well, fit and healthy in a natural way using products without side effects or as little side effects as possible.

So Ulrich Sommer knows both sides of the coin – the pharmaceutical way of healing and the natural way. Knowing what he knew there was no choice other than to make the change to more natural methods of healing, and he never looked back.

"Mr. Sommer, when you were a pharmacist, did you also sell medications promoted by the pharmaceutical industry?"

Ulrich Sommer: "Of course, that's mainly what a pharmacist does, and by law he is required to do so. However, from the very beginning, when I was asked, I always consulted toward natural healing."

"Why is that?"

Ulrich Sommer: "I had problems with my own body so I tried every possible way to improve my own body conditions and strengthen the immune system."

"Was there a point you developed an antipathy against normal drugs or medications?"

Ulrich Sommer: "I wouldn't say antipathy. But I became disillusioned when I once tried a drug for myself. It was a drug sold over the counter at that time to improve mood and self esteem, quite popular; later it became a prescription drug."

"Why did you take it and what were the effects?"

Ulrich Sommer: "I was apprehensive about my examinations coming up. I took the drug to help it. At first I felt wonderful. What this medication or drug actually did was alter reality. Therefore I was unable to solve problems and I flunked every test. Catastrophic! And I took that drug only a few times. So I decided never to take those types of medication again. Without this drug, I never flunked a test afterwards and passed the whole examination without difficulties."

"What were the exact side effects of this medication?"

Ulrich Sommer: "I would say it hindered my ability to compute analytically, the exact thing I needed to pass my exam."

"Nevertheless, you sold a lot of medications from the pharmaceutical industry to customers when you were a pharmacist. What were your experiences there?"

Ulrich Sommer: "I became increasingly hesitant to dispense these products, asking myself, 'What am I doing here? Should I say something and discourage the patient from taking those?' And when possible I tried to direct the patient towards less invasive medications. However the result was that the patient came back from the doctor who opposed my recommendation. So there was definitely a conflict."

"What was your experience with customers who were sold hard medications, like sleeping pills or painkillers?"

Ulrich Sommer: "I observed that patients who were taking these medications tend to develop a dependency, especially when alcohol was involved."

"Nevertheless, what were your thoughts as you sold drugs to your customers?"

Ulrich Sommer: "I had conflicting thoughts: on one hand I was trained as a pharmacist and on the other hand I observed the effects of the drugs."

"How many customers did you have as an apothecary?"

Ulrich Sommer: "Several thousands."

"What happened to those customers or some of those customers?"

Ulrich Sommer: "They came in good faith to receive help for their specific condition and often after receiving the prescription to 'handle' the condition were not only not improved but also presented with an additional health problem which required another drug. This can easily be prevented if one would take the time to read the instruction leaflets listing all the potential side effects of most prescription drugs. I saw people who started out with a light problem ending up with severe conditions and even death."

"What did you think while seeing all this?"

Ulrich Sommer: "I thought, it must be possible to treat these individuals successfully with medicines that do not have these side effects. Doctors should not be afraid to lose business. They should treat towards wellness, not just put a 'bandage' on the symptoms. Long term, they would have healthy 'customers' with a considerably longer life."

"What were the worst effects you could see; which medications were the most dangerous ones?"

Ulrich Sommer: "Tranquilizers and so called psychotropic drugs without doubt, then sleeping pills, painkillers."

"In simplified words, how would you describe the effects of those medications?"

Ulrich Sommer: "It appears in the beginning, that those medications have a kind of protective effect. What really happens is the patient is inhibited from facing reality. Can he solve his problems this way? Absolutely not. The patient further declines, both physically and emotionally by the influence of these chemicals. He feels the effects of the environment are not as strong as before. So one feels it helps. The life force however, or élan vital, like the French philosopher Henry Bergson called it, gets weaker."

"What happens with those patients usually?"

Ulrich Sommer: "When they discontinue the use of the drug, withdrawal symptoms set in. This forces them to continue taking the medications so it ends with a dependency on the drug with the liability of encountering devastating side effects."

"Besides the psychotropic drugs, sleeping pills, and pain pills, what other drugs have the most side effects?"

Ulrich Sommer: "The medications that stop the growth of cells, such as the cancer therapies (chemotherapy), have disastrous side effects. And another is the misuse of antibiotics. In the seventies, one would take an antibiotic medication for practically every little cold. But after a while, when you receive too many antibiotics, the body becomes less resistant against bacteria. Today, more and more complex antibiotics have to be given in order to be effective. Too many antibiotics can have a host of side effects and the whole immune system can become suppressed after a while."

"If you look at all those existing pharmaceutical products, what percentage, in your evaluation, are for the birds or even harmful? And are there pharmaceutical products which are worthwhile taking?"

Ulrich Sommer: “First I must say it is not possible to give a reliable estimate due to the vast amount of drugs that are today on the market. The number has increased exponentially since my days as a pharmacist. There are products which are necessary and are valuable. The majority I´m afraid are not necessary and too often harmful.”

“Give us an example of ‘good drugs.’”

Ulrich Sommer: “There are definitely situations where antibiotics and painkillers are life saving. If you have a heart attack, a tranquilizer, temporarily given, could save your life. Immune suppressants are vital when you undergo a transplant.”

“However, when only a small percentage of all those medications are worthwhile, what about the rest? It is for the birds? Or even worse, is it dangerous?”

Ulrich Sommer: “Instead of many thousands of products, one could possibly achieve the same results with just a few hundred. Too many products are with too little positive effect and rather harmful, and could and should be eliminated.”

“What is the biggest mistake in the computation of the pharmaceutical industry?”

Ulrich Sommer: “How they can increase their market share and how they can make more profit. Which is economically correct? But is it also the optimum benefit for the patients, for the general health of our society, for mankind? Further the obsession to treat the symptoms with chemical compounds rather than working with natural substances. And also trying to treat one isolated organ rather than taking a holistic approach.”

"Didn't you try as a pharmacist to cooperate directly with some doctors and offer them better medications – plant-based medications?"

Ulrich Sommer: "In fact, I did. But it was not very successful. I observed that there was rather the intention or tendency to treat the patient's symptoms than finding the real cause and making the patient well. This gives you the effect that the patient must return to the doctor again and again endlessly. More viable for the doctor and the pharmacist – but on the long run...?"

"What percentage of the doctors really like to help?"

Ulrich Sommer: "That is a very good question. I don't know. I think that originally many of the doctors wanted to help. I think in the beginning, most doctors have the best intentions. However they need to survive "in the system.""

"How do you evaluate the pharmaceutical industry as a whole?"

Ulrich Sommer: "Certainly there have been and will continue to be benefits for society with the proper use of specific drugs. However drugs become increasingly abused to the detriment of society as a whole. For example, drugging children because of their learning disabilities due to false labeling by psychiatrists. It has been documented that diseases are artificially created so that drugs can be marketed on a larger scale."

"What is the pharmaceutical drug-cartel actually doing to protect their profits?"

Ulrich Sommer: “First of all, you see more and more laws and regulations. Natural products or plant based or biological products are increasingly forbidden. The admission and the concession of good products is hindered or slowed down for obvious reasons. In addition, the industry tries to buy those other biologically oriented firms wholesale, so that they can make the profits and run them their way. Aside from that, some of the big pharmaceutical companies already run parallel programs and look into this new market that wants plant-based or biological products. In each case, it is always about markets, markets, markets.”

“Can one refer to the pharmaceutical industry as a cartel today? Is that expression correct?”

Ulrich Sommer: “Per definition a cartel is an association of manufacturers or suppliers formed to maintain high prices and restrict competition. I think it is rather obvious how that definition applies.”

“What is the true intention of the pharmaceutical drug cartel?”

Ulrich Sommer: “For example there is the Codex Alimentarius. It would be too elaborate to get into detail about the Codex at this point. One of the purposes of this “Codex” appears to be to eliminate, with the help of the lawmakers, smaller manufacturers and suppliers of nutritional supplements so that the pharmaceutical industry can take over the market. Another one is most certainly the increase of their market by creating and selling more and more drugs.”

“What are the creation costs of those medications?”

Ulrich Sommer: "I don't know their calculations. But a lot of drugs appear to be quite profitable if one compares the actual cost of the chemical with the price of the end product."

"What are the tactics and strategies against the natural products?"

Ulrich Sommer: "There are more and more restrictions on nutritional supplements. Restrictions originally were very different from country to country. Today there is a tendency towards globalization, which seeks to include countries that had fewer restrictions like The Netherlands, England and the United States. In the USA there are even efforts to forbid giving testimonials. Testimonials one day will be permitted to print only when backed by exact studies – double blind studies – which are very expensive and time-consuming and sometimes nearly impossible. There is a tendency to make it harder and harder to sell other products than those of the pharmaceutical industry."

"How is the pharmacist dependent upon the pharmaceutical industry?"

Ulrich Sommer: "As retailer, the pharmacist is at the end of the supplier chain as he purchases products from the wholesale merchant. The wholesaler buys from pharmaceutical companies. Thus the pharmacist has very little influence on prices and sales and about 80% of his turnover comes from prescription drugs which require the prescription of the doctor."

"And the doctors themselves are dependent upon the pharmaceutical industry?"

Ulrich Sommer: "Yes, for the evaluation of the drug. It appears that the majority of doctors trust that drugs are as safe as they are promoted. There are shows, events and meetings to launch new products on the market. The target group is the doctor. In the end, the pharmacy gets the smaller part of business; the big business is between the doctors and the pharmaceutical industry."

"Can the doctor evaluate a new prescription drug easily?"

Ulrich Sommer: "Theoretically yes, what I observed was that doctors have hardly the time to look into everything when it comes to a new prescription drug. They get lectures by representatives of the pharmaceutical industry and usually believe their reports."

"How do the pharmaceutical companies ensure that they stay on top of the game?"

Ulrich Sommer: "By using lobbyists to influence politicians, parliaments, governments internationally."

"In theory, how could the apothecaries free themselves from the pharmaceutical industry?"

Ulrich Sommer: "The Pharmaceutical Industry, doctors and pharmacies all depend on each other. Their relationship needs to be more balanced and must include the benefits of the patient, society and mankind. The key is with the doctors as they are writing the prescriptions. Finally the patient must be educated as to the effects of the medications he is taking. And a step before that would be to have a good education in health and nutrition so he would not get into the position in the first place to need the doctor or the pharmacist."

"So in the end it does NOT boil down to the politician and the law?"

Ulrich Sommer: "Ideally not."

"Mr. Sommer, thank you for the interview."

Ulrich Sommer: "My pleasure!"

3. DRUGS FOR THE OLD AND THE ELDERLY

Before we go into actual side effects, let us first look into the facts and nothing but facts.

The book, which doctors most often use in reviewing drugs, is called the *Physicians' Desk Reference*, often referred to as *PDR*. The 2008 edition is the 62nd edition (a new one comes out every year) and is over *3,500* pages long.[58] The American drug *formulary*[59] is enormous which leads one to wonder how doctors can safely dispense from such a huge source of drugs, and yet the American drug arsenal is viewed as a sort of cornucopia[60] of health care solutions.

The poly-pharmaceutical geriatric market is a gold mine for the drug industry. "Poly" means *many*. "Pharmaceutical" means something from the *pharmacy*: a drug. "Geriatric" means *elderly or old*. A remarkable thing has occurred in American society. Since people are living longer and longer, a new category has come into modern health usage. If a person is between 55 and 65, he is said to be "older." "Elderly" doesn't kick in until a person is over 65. Thus the elderly and the older are an enormous market for the drug industry. According to the *United States Census bureau,* the USA has a population of 35 million people aged 65 and over. This market has been increasing and has, in fact, increased 12% since the 1990 census.[61] With the baby boomers becoming old, it is likely that this section of the population will grow at an even higher rate in the next census. In 2000, 18.4 million people were 65 to 74 years old. This was slightly more than half of the population over the age of 65.

58 PDR https://www.pdrbookstore.com/Default.asp?

59 Formulary: the entire list of drugs available to the physician

60 Cornucopia: horn of plenty

61 United States Census Bureau, http://www.census.gov/prod/2001pubs/c2kbr01-10.pdf

Advancing age brings with it degeneration of the body. While many problems can be avoided or delayed through a healthy lifestyle, it is nonetheless a fact that the elderly need and use more health care than any other age group. Since much of the elderly health market is served by doctors of medicine (M.D.'s) and osteopathy[62] (D.O.'s), the use of prescription drugs among the elderly is greatest compared to all other age groups. An *osteopath* is virtually identical to a medical doctor in that he can perform surgery and can prescribe any drug in the pharmacy. He is different in that he emphasizes the treatment of medical disorders through the manipulation and management of the bones, joints and muscles.[63] In actual practice, D.O.'s rarely manipulate patients for relief.

Because of the various infirmities and illnesses associated with advancing age, the elderly use drugs in extensive quantities. The medications are prescribed for high blood pressure, arthritis, lung conditions, nerve disorders, cancer, heart disease and a host of other illnesses. A study at *Duke University Medical Center* has found that, while the elderly consist of less than 15% of the total population, they consume about one-third of all prescription drugs.[64] Thus the elderly constitute a major market for the American pharmaceutical industry. The twelve largest drug companies have total annual revenue of $291.2 billion.[65] The portion attributable to the elderly market is $97.1 billion dollars.

The cost of the drugs has been escalating for many years. The 30 most frequently prescribed drugs for the elderly are all fairly newly developed. The FDA approved 26 of the drugs since the year 2000. When averaged out, the annual increase in the costs of these drugs is more than 3.5 times the rate of inflation. The average cost of the

---

62 Osteopathy: a system of medicine based on the theory that many diseases are caused by incorrect alignments of bones, ligaments, and muscles, and that correcting these through manipulation can cure the problems. It is often effective in treating joint and muscle disorders. MSN Encarta Online Dictionary

63 *MSN Encarta Online Dictionary.* http://encarta.msn.com/dictionary_/osteopathy.html

64 Lesley H.Curtis, Ph.D.,Duke University Medical Center, Durham, N.C.

65 *Wall Street Journal,* May 21, 2004 for the year 2003

top 30 drugs from January 2003 to January 2004 was 6.5%. During the same period, the rate of inflation in the USA economy was 1.5%. The profits generated from this target group are increasing at more than 2.5 times the annual rise in the rate of inflation. No other industry has profit performances that exceed these figures.

Even since 1999, it is interesting to see the difference in cost per year for the consumer. According to AARP, a consumer using Ambien pays $900 a year more at the end of 2006 that he did in 1999. He would pay more than $500 more per year for Plavix and the same for Zocor. Using Celebrex, he would've paid $300 more per year and $100 more per year for Toprol. Outrageous! This is so many more times the cost of living.[66]

In the following chart are listed the biggest selling drugs used by the elderly.[67]

Brand Name	Strength	Therapeutic Category	Marketer	2004 Cost/year	2006 Cost/year
Ambien	5 mg	Anticonvulsant and Muscle Relaxant for Insomnia	Aventis	$350	$922
Plavix	75 mg	Anti-platelet Agent	BMS	$425	$511
Zocor	20 mg	Lipid[68] Lowering Agent	Merck	$350	$485
Celebrex	200 mg	Anti/Inflammatory Beta-blocker for	Pfizer	$175	$281
Toprol	50 mg	Angina for angina and hypertension	Astra Zeneca	$75	$105

66 TRENDS IN MANUFACTURER PRICES OF BRAND-NAME PRESCRIPTION DRUGS USED BY OLDER AMERICANS—2006 YEAR-END UPDATE – http://assets.aarp.org/rgcenter/health/dd154_drugprices.pdf

67 Taken from a chart prepared by the AARP Public Policy Institute and the *PRIME* Institute, University of Minnesota, based on data from Medi-Span Price-Chek PC (Indianapolis, IN: Wolters Kluwer Health Inc., February 2007). http://assets.aarp.org/rgcenter/health/dd154_drugprices.pdf

68 A *lipid* is a fatty substance in the blood. The lipid-lowering drug reduces cholesterol. A *platelet* is a component of blood. The *anti-platelet* drug prevents blood clots. *Osteoporosis* is a disease in which bones become brittle and likely to break. By keeping calcium out of the heart and blood vessel cells, the cells relax and chest pain and high blood pressure are controlled. A *gastrointestinal agent* controls stomach and bowel discomfort.

The figures under the yearly columns show the increase in the average annual wholesale price for these medications.[69]

Medicare is a major component of elderly health care. It is a federal health insurance program for people over the age of 65.[70] There are 39 million people on the *Medicare* program. *Medicare* does not pay for most prescription drug costs; however, its expenditures for drugs are significant. In 2003, it spent over $10.5 billion on pharmaceuticals for the elderly.[71] AARP,[72] an advocacy group for the elderly, issued a report that analyzed drug prices for 197 of the medications most often used by patients over 65 years of age. It found that there was an overall increase of 3.4% in the first three months of 2004. It confirmed the fact that the drug-price increases are out pacing inflation by more than two-fold. Even the rate of increase is increasing. The rate of increase for 2003 was 6.9%. This increase in profits is extraordinary considering that there was actually a drop in inflation during 2002 and only a slight increase in 2003.[73] In 2004, the prices rose 6%, nearly twice the general inflation rate that was 3.6%.[74] Since then, after 2005 there was a slight drop of 6%, but by 2006 that had gone up to 6.2%. But this is still nearly double the rate of increase of inflation, which is currently at 3.2%.[75]

---

69 Source: AARP Public Policy Institute. TRENDS IN MANUFACTURER PRICES OF BRAND-NAME PRESCRIPTION DRUGS USED BY OLDER AMERICANS – 2006 YEAR-END UPDATE: http://assets.aarp.org/rgcenter/health/dd154_drugprices.pdf

70 While the vast majority of people in the program are the elderly, it also serves the disabled and, oddly, those with end-stage kidney disease. The latter was added because a USA lawmaker had a daughter with an end-stage kidney disease.

71 *Medicare and Prescription Drug Costs-Part II*, http://www.therubins.com/medicare/drugcost2.htm

72 AARP: American Association of Retired Persons

73 AARP. http://Assets.aarp.org/rgcenter/post-import/2004_06_drugprices.pdf

74 AARP. http://Assets.aarp.org/rgcenter/post-import/dd112_brand_drugs.pdf

75 See footnote at 69.

MEDICARE AND MEDICAID

Medicare prescriptions underwent new changes in January of 2006. Medicaid is a health insurance program for low-income seniors and others. Matching funds for drugs under *Medicaid* is no longer available in the new plan. *Medicare* is offering a new drug benefit, called *Medicare* Part D. Subsidy funds are available to help the elderly poor buy drugs. After the *Medicare - Medicaid* revision the prices of 20 most common prescription drugs was hiked up by an average of 3.7%. This goes to show that, except for some incremental chipping, federal efforts to curb pharmaceutical expense have not been successful historically. The prices of drugs for the elderly are expected to continue to rise.[76]

Nearly nine out of every ten Medicare beneficiaries fill at least one prescription annually. According to a Congressional Budget Office report, the average elderly patient spends $860 per year for prescription drugs. This expenditure is more than what the average elderly person spends for doctors, medical supplies and vision expenses.[77]

Approximately 40% of all Medicare patients lack coverage for prescription drug coverage. A supplemental drug insurance does exist to cover some of the *Medicare* elderly. AARP has taken the position that there is a risk of that coverage being lost. To support this position, AARP points out that the number of companies offering supplemental drug coverage to its retirees has dropped 7% from 1997 to 2001. Also, there has been a drop of 15% in drug coverage plans to the elderly. Most plans now cover only generic drugs. Co-pays for *Medigap* policies (policies designed to cover medical expenses not covered by Medicare) are tending not to cover drug costs, or have higher deductibles and less coverage.[78] The focus of the AARP lobby is to get the government to pay more for drugs for

---

76 Kathy Jones, "Drug Prices Increase Under Part D Plan," *Families USA*, June 21, 2006

77 AARP, http://www.aarp.org/research/health/drugs/aresearch-import-656-DD77.html

78 http://www.aarp.org/research/health/drugs/aresearch-import-656-DD77.html

the elderly and to encourage government oversight and control of drug pricing. In summary, the net effect of this is:

Name of Drug	What it treats	Cost for 1-year supply
Lipitor	Cholesterol control	$871
Novasc	A calcium channel blocker	$549
Fosamax	Bone density	$894
Prilosec (20 mg)	Anti-ulcer	$1,684
Celebrex	Rheumatoid Arthritis	$2,102[79]

In addition, here are some more facts:

FACT: The average American over the age of 75 takes more than 11 drugs.

FACT: More and more potential new drugs are in development for the elderly.

FACT: Primary Care Physicians account for 53% of the prescription.

FACT: Three of the top ten drugs for the elderly are medications used to treat mood problems and depressions.[80]

And let us repeat the already established facts:

FACT: The elderly are the largest group of prescription drug consumers.

FACT: The cost of drugs to the elderly is increasing faster than the rate of inflation.

FACT: It is expected to maintain this increase.

FACT: Efforts to control prescription drug costs have not been successful.

FACT: The projected drug savings costs, if any, for Medicare Part D are unknown.

79 Source: information contained in the report "Enough to Make Your Sick: Prescription Drug Prices for the Elderly" from *Families USA*

80 http://www.therubins.com/geninfo/eldpresc.htm

VIAGRA, CONTINUED

So far we just discussed the money. But we didn't talk about the side effects of all those drugs. So let's pick out just a few examples. And let us continue with our '*Viagra* Story' originally designed for the elderly. Because the fact is, we didn't even mention one tenth of the truth about Viagra. So let's take a closer look.

One problem for the elderly population is the lessening sex-drive. Impotence, erectile dysfunctions, and less sexual interest are normal with age. We already spoke of the victory that Viagra represents in terms of money: the billions of dollars they made. As a result, Pfizer's shares soared from $45 to $115 in 2004. Viagra substitutes came on the market: herbal Viagra, cheap Viagra, Viagra online, Viagra alternatives, you name it. Viagra, originally approved as an impotence pill by the Food and Drug Administration (FDA) in 1998, isn't only used today by people with erectile dysfunctions; one can find it in sex shops and in marital-aid catalogues. It is a chic, fashion pill; people even pretended to have erectile problems to get Viagra prescriptions. The main target, being the elderly population, expanded like mad with the support of the media, knowing that with sex you can attract viewers, listeners and readers. However, Viagra was an unbelievable success – and this despite the side effects.

We mentioned previously that the package insert is 18 pages long. The cardio-vascular patient using Viagra and engaging in sex has a higher risk for heart attack. But this is only part of the picture, so let's look more closely at this pill that allegedly provides us with a wonderful new world.

In point of fact, serious problems occurred during the testing of *Sildenafil - Viagra*. This information was not readily available to the general public and was only made available by the Federal Drug Administration (FDA) after being served with an official demand under the *Freedom of Information Act.*[81] The FDA says that there is no known direct link between the deaths and Viagra. And yet there were 16 fatal cases in this first release.

---

81 http://junkscience.com/news2/viagra4.htm

Here are the fatalities that occurred during testing, the ages ranging from 48 to 80. The 80-year-old man died while having sex. The 48-year-old man experienced chests pains during the sex act. He was taken to a hospital where he died in the emergency room some hours later. Seven of these 16 cases died after the sex act. Most of the group had other health related problems including hypertension (dangerously high blood pressure), heart disease and diabetes. The cause of death was usually attributed to heart disease. Some of the men had poly-pharmaceutical problems including the administration of nitrates (including nitroglycerin) that are dangerous when taken with Sildenafil. The FDA would not say that there were any previously unidentified dangers related to the use of Viagra. An FDA spokesperson, Lorrie McHugh, was quoted as saying, "We continue to believe the drug is safe, when used by appropriate patients."[82]

Following the trials, there were more cases of reported deaths issued by the FDA. In August of 1998, just four months after the drug was released, 69 more deaths were reported. The agency did not feel that these deaths presented a problem. Since, at this time, over 3.6 million prescriptions had been written, the number of deaths was considered to be small. In this second batch of deaths, the FDA revealed that 18 of the patients died while having sex or just afterward. In seven other cases leading to death, symptoms appeared within five hours of the sex act. The deaths are divided into 46 cardiovascular events, 2 strokes and 21 of unknown causes. The ranges of the dead were from 29 to 87, while the median age was 64. Twelve cases involved adverse poly-pharmaceuticals, and 51 of the 69 had other risk factors including heart disease, smoking, obesity and high blood pressure.[83]

It is widely believed that the deaths from Viagra are greatly under-reported. If an older person, who does not regularly engage in sex, suddenly begins having vigorous sexual intercourse, the result is a potentially serious strain on the heart. Often, the surviving sex

82 http://www.cnn.com/HEALTH/9805/22/viagra.patients/index.html

83 http://www.sddt.com/News/article.cfm?SourceCode=19980826fe

partner is reluctant to report that the death occurred during the sex act. Thus, many Viagra related deaths might be reported as a heart attack without further explanation or examination.

Another factor, which results in under-reporting of side effects, is that there are many cases in which the drug is taken by those other than the ones for whom it was prescribed. We mentioned that already. It turns out that 43% of women suffer from sexual dysfunction, a number greater than their male counterparts. Dr. Myron Murdoch, a urology professor at George Washington Medical School has also said that Viagra can restore sexual functioning.[84] Pfizer even conducted testing over a period of *eight years* to show that Viagra is good for women. They were unable to prove correlation largely because female sex problems are often due to *emotions*, unlike men whose problem is lack of blood flow to achieve an erection. Pfizer gave up on the trials for women, but many of them still use it. A black market has been established and sales of the drug to women are flourishing. Additionally, the women get the drug from their sexual partners who have legitimate prescriptions.[85]

Another black market public that results in under-reporting is that involving young men and women who attend rave clubs. The men take a drug called *Sextasy*, which is a combination of the street drug *ecstasy* and Viagra.[86] Since the drug ecstasy acts as a un-inhibitor, the result is a widely promiscuous course of behavior with its attendant problems in risky sexual behavior. The drug is readily available although it is supposed to be sold only with a doctor's prescription, through pharmacies for $8-10 per pill. It is currently obtainable easily over the Internet. The black-market rate has run from $25 to $30.[87] There is evidence to suggest that young healthy men are at risk to more than just sexually transmitted disease with the use of Viagra. Researchers at the *Cedars-Sinai Medical Center*

84 Christopher Gearon, "The Search for a Female Viagra," *Discovery*, http://health.discovery.com/centers/womens/viagra/viagra.html

85 Ibid.

86 ABC News, reported by BLTC, http://mdma.net/sexstasy

87 Karen S. Petersen, *USA Today*, March 21, 2001, http://www.usatoday.com/news/health/2001-03-21-viagra-abuse.htm

in Los Angeles analyzed various post-marketing adverse event reports that were filed with the Federal Drug Administration by the Pfizer Corporation. Unlike the elderly men with other adverse health factors, the new data showed that Viagra is present in cases of heart attacks in younger men. Most of the reported deaths, which occurred within a few hours of taking the drug, were of men under the age of 65 who:

- Had no reported heart conditions;
- Had the standard, prescribed dose.

The epidemiologists at Cedars-Sinai stated that there "appears to be a high number of deaths and serious cardiovascular events associated with the use of Viagra." The study was presented at a meeting of the *American College of Cardiologists* in Anaheim, California. There were 1,473 major adverse events analyzed in the Viagra FDA report. Of these, deaths occurred in 522 cases. Most of the deaths occurred from adverse cardiovascular events. The senior author, Dr. Sinjay Kaul, found that 70% of the fatalities were associated with a 50-milligram dose, the standard Viagra Dose. The study confirmed that the use of nitrates in conjunction with Viagra is a deadly combination. But the analysis showed that 88% of the deaths involved people who were not using any nitrates. This leads health investigators "to speculate whether there are some susceptible individuals who don't need nitrates to unmask the harmful effects of Viagra."[88] As of September 2001, 16 million men had taken Viagra. Sales were $1.5 billion per year. Six hundred and forty deaths were reported.[89] This is evidence that the number of deaths associated with Viagra exceeded that of other drugs that have been recalled. A number of non-fatal strokes have been associated with the use of the drug. The adverse information produced in the post-marketing-effect reports were not disclosed to the consumer. The insert warnings are inadequate and should be modified.

---

88 "Viagra May Cause Heart Attack Deaths In Younger Men With No heart Problems, Study Finds," *PSA Rising Magazine*, May 14, 2000, http://psa-rising.com/medicalpike/vaigracardiodeaths031500.htm

89 *Future*, http://www.globalchange.com/viagranews2.htm

ASPIRIN, CONTINUED

Let us continue the story about aspirin. Aspirin is not necessarily typical for the elderly population, but the *side effects* show up to a large degree in that group.

Did you know that *aspirin* use is linked with pancreatic cancer? (The pancreas is a large gland behind the stomach that aids in digestion and secretes insulin.) Fourteen aspirins a week increases the risk for pancreatic cancer by 86%, 6 – 13 a week still 41% bolstered risk and 1 – 3, 11% elevated risk. Adverse drug reactions (ADR) are a long term, huge problem in Great Britain, for example, and account for 1 in 16 hospital admissions.[90]

Heavy use of pain medication harms kidneys; heavy use of aspirins (or acetaminophen) is associated with a recently discovered condition affecting people with irreversible kidney failure. The condition is known as sick (small, indented and calcified) kidneys.

MORE ON OSTEOPOROSIS

Again the simple definition: The term *porosia* simply indicates a *porous* condition; *osteo* points to the *bones.* Older men and women are not as strong as younger people. This includes the bones. But *osteoporosis* points to an actual disease. The bones become porous and brittle because of a loss of calcium. But here we are. Of course that provides the pharmaceutical industry with a new market. Hurrah! Instead of treating people simply with calcium combined with magnesium, one can create a multi-billion-dollar business. Instead of teaching people in which foods one can find lots of calcium, one can invent a pill, with an exclusive patent, and bingo.

90 Note: ADR increases exponentially with 4 or more medications. In the USA, 2.8 billion prescriptions were filled in 2000, which means about 10 prescriptions for every person in the United States. Adverse drug reactions kill over 100,000 plus Americans every year. Adverse drug reactions are already the No. 4 killer in the USA after heart disease, cancer and stroke.

As a note here, proper exercise and nutrition help to build and maintain strong bones and in addition to calcium intake, vitamin D is essential. The cost of taking 1200-1500 mg of calcium and 400-800 IU of vitamin D daily would cost only about $3.60 a month.

Another method consists of putting people onto hormone therapy. And yes, hormones do have an influence on the bones; hormones are an issue. So what is the best thing to do in the eyes of a pharmaceutical executive? The best thing to do is to invent a "Hormone Replacement Therapy" (HRT), get some "scientists" (paid by the pharmaceutical industry of course) stating how effective HRT is and then advertise it like crazy.

Hormones and "Hormone Replacement Therapy" (HRT) became popular, despite the horrible side effects that were documented well. Here are the facts. The latest study on HRT and osteoporosis shows that women, following the usual recommendation to take the drug for ten years upon the start of menopause, are not protected from brittle bone disease any more than those women who have never taken the drug at all!

The bad effect of "Hormone Replacement Therapy" (HRT) far outweighs the benefits. Women taking HRT have a significantly higher likelihood of a vast array of other diseases, as well as death, compared with those not taking the medications. HRT use raises the risk of cardiovascular disease by 78%. HRT even raises a woman's chance to develop asthma.

One large-scale review of 31 studies on osteoporosis concluded that estrogen (a female sex hormone) didn't have any significant benefit in slowing the onset of osteoporosis. Too bad! But don't think for a second the pharmaceutical industry will give up. There is a market here, a huge market. And one isn't pretending to be a prophet saying that there will be all kinds of other pills and therapies in the next ten, twenty years.

THE CHOLESTEROL DEBATE

We mentioned earlier about a strategy, to define new risk factors, make them public, develop a pill, and earn a hell of a lot of money with it. The debate of the century about risk factor is of course the famous cholesterol, the "bad cholesterol."

Some factors first: We need cholesterol for every cell, for digestion, for nerves, for brain, skin, bones and heart muscle. Cholesterol is ABSOLUTELY NECESSARY, in other words. Without enough cholesterol, ramifications such as obesity, digestion problems, impotence, blood pressure problems and even emotional problems show up. In 1990, cholesterol was assigned the role of the culprit for cardiovascular diseases, stroke and cardiac infarction. Some experts started to differentiate between HDL (high-density lipo-protein) or "good" cholesterol and LDL (low-density lipo-protein or "bad" cholesterol. A *lipo-protein*, simply spoken, is a combination of *protein* and *lipids*, pointing to fat/cholesterol. Basically, HDL contains another type of protein as LDL. LDL or "bad" cholesterol is what plugs up the blood vessel walls. Nutritionists (like Judith A. De Cava),[91] doctors (like Lynne McTaggart)[92] and professors (like George V. Mann), and Professors of Medicine & Biochemistry, *Vanderbilt University*, looked closer into the debate regarding good and bad cholesterol.

We don't want to stress the reader's patience with scientific arguments, but Prof. George V. Mann simply stated that "saturated" fat and cholesterol in the diet are *not* the cause of coronary heart disease. That myth is the greatest scientific deception of this century – perhaps of any century.[93] The renowned author, De Cava, simply talks about the "Cholesterol Conspiracy"[94] as the "most inaccurate

91 Judith A. De Cava, *Cholesterol, Facts & Fantasies*, (Centerville, Massachusetts, 1994)

92 Lynne McTaggart, *What Doctors Don't Tell You*, (New York: Harper Collins, 2002)

93 Quotation found by Judith A. De Cava, p. 3

94 De Cava, p. 6

test,"[95] and points to the "French paradox." French men eat LOTS of fat/cholesterol, and the death rate from heart diseases in France is lower than in USA (France, 95 out of 100,000 men versus the USA, 256 out of 100,000 men). De Cava also talks about the longest living people in Europe (people in the Island of Crete) who eat fat, fat, fat and get as old as the Japanese people. She quotes scientific inquires and ends with, "There is no question that the cholesterol program… benefits three powerful groups in our society to the tune of literally billions of dollars. These three are the medical professions, the pharmaceutical industry and the food companies."[96]

However, the truth remains unchallenged: millions and millions of prescriptions to lower cholesterol are written every year in the USA (and in other countries as well). The cholesterol-lowering drugs are big business. In fact, it is the biggest and most wonderful business one can imagine. On the other hand, the side effects of those drugs are also "well documented."

Here are just some side effects:

- Lowering cholesterol (allegedly the cause of hardening arteries) may *increase* the risk factors of death by stroke.
- And certain cholesterol drugs may increase the risk of *cancer* by 1/3.
- Other evidence has shown a greater risk of *suicide*! A number of large-scale studies showed that patients on low cholesterol diets or drugs were more likely to die from violent deaths, including suicide, then those eating what they want.
- One study in a geriatric unit in Italy found that among older people the risk of *depression* was highest among those with the lowest cholesterol concentration. The proof for all those side effects was given by Lynne McTaggart in her already quoted book "What Doctors Don't Tell You."

95 De Cava, p. 6

96 De Cava, p. 40, De Cava quoting Lynne Mc Taggart

So to reiterate the important information:

- The bad-cholesterol debate brought billions of dollars into the pocket of the pharmaceutical industry.
- Quite horrifying side effects are documented.

The scientific findings about "bad cholesterol" are, to say the least, controversial.

THE PRESCRIPTION DILEMMA

To recapitulate, the pharmaceutical industry earns billions of dollars from the old and the elderly. But the side effects of some medications are horrifying. Nevertheless, a stupid belief in the drug – the Almighty Drug – continues to plague us. And we haven't even mentioned a much greater danger we face today, when it comes to drugs. With all this money being spent to create a cornucopia of drugs, how can a doctor insure the safety of his patients?

When the authors were young, a trip to the doctor for a medical problem would result in the doctor studying the patient, poking and prodding, asking questions, and then he would prescribe a medicine which he thought was best for the patient's problem. Times have changed.

Today's elderly drug consumer is barraged with advertising from drug companies. The art is glossy and expensive. The TV spots are catchy, pithy and sometimes humorous. The pitch is always the same: "Ask your doctor if Widgetal® is for you."[97] This direct promotion is driving people into the physician's office and driving up the sale of prescription medicine. The consumer is encouraged to take more, and more, prescription drugs. Poly-pharmaceutical (multiple prescriptions) use is on the rise. Since, as a person ages, he or she acquires more and more physical problems, the tendency is to take more and more medications. About 80% of the elderly suffer from one chronic condition or another. More than 50% of

97 Widgetal®: a made-up name for a drug. A "widget" is a mythical thing used for discussion in college business classes.

them have two or more chronic diseases.[98] (We define "chronic" as lasting over a long period of time, as opposed to "acute," which means of a limited sharp duration.)

Poly-pharmacy is defined as the concurrent use of multiple prescription medications. It can occur at any age level, but it is most prevalent among the elderly. There have been several studies that find that patients aged 65 and over will have an average of two to six prescribed medications and 1 to 3.4 non-prescribed medications. The elderly tend to use these multiple medications on a regular, ongoing basis. The issue was highlighted in a *Healthy People 2000* white paper.[99]

In 1999, a physician survey found that 66% of all doctor visits resulted in prescriptions being written. This was an increase of 5% from the preceding year. Of 756 million visits in the study, drugs were prescribed 501 million times. Multiple issued prescriptions jumped from 107 per 100 visits to 146 prescriptions per 100 visits. Most of the multiple prescriptions were written for the elderly. Catharine W. Burt, chief of ambulatory care statistics at *the National Center for Health Statistics*, who administered the study, stated that the increase in prescribing is "...a lot more than we would have expected just from the aging of the population." The increase was largely attributed to aggressive marketing by the drug companies. Heavily advertised drugs tended to be in the top twenty most prescribed drugs. Some good news came from the study. Prescriptions for antibiotics are down.[100]

There is little research on the safety and effectiveness of mixing multiple medications in a single patient. In fact, there is no body of pharmacology capable of making such a study. Epidemiologists (those who study health intervention attributes) may be able to create an effective way to study it, but it would be impeded or stopped by

---

98 Pamela D. Larson and Janice L. Hoot Martin, "Polypharmacy and Elderly Patients," *AORN JOURNAL,* March 1999. Reported at http://www.findarticles.com/p/articles/mi_m0FSL/is_3_69/ai_54216921

99 Larson and Martin, Ibid.

100 Over-prescription of antibiotics has been blamed for the build up of drug resistant strains of bacteria. Ibid.

the fact that there are so many different ways to *shake and bake* the drug mixes that it would be hard to find the consistently defined test groups (those who get the drug cocktails) and control groups (those who get the sugar pills).[101]

Here is a chilling analogy. A scientist working in a laboratory would never randomly mix eight or more different chemicals in a test tube without studying the projected effect of the chemicals. "Thus, when an elderly patient is prescribed eight to ten medications concurrently, it is impossible to predict the outcome."[102] Studies show that the elderly take over 30% of all medications prescribed.[103] There is an attitude prevalent among elderly patients (and among patients in general), that if the doctor does not give the patient a prescription, the doctor's visit was a failure.[104]

All drugs have side effects. When the drugs are taken together, it opens the door to a host of new side effects. For example, one case that one of the authors is familiar with, involved an old woman who was being treated for cancer, hypertension and diabetes. She described the side effect as "being on fire" and was quite distressed. The fiery feeling was not a listed side effect of any one drug and was actually a new side effect of the poly-pharmaceutical treatment. These case studies are often dismissed as "anecdotal" and without proof by the FDA and the drug companies. This is true. To prove it, you would have to treat lots of patients with the drug cocktail and have lots of non-treated patients (the placebo or sugar pill group) with which to compare them. This would be unethical.

Research has shown that the greater the number of drugs taken by an elderly patient, the more likely she or he is to have a harmful side effect of the drugs.[105] This is called a "risk factor,"

101 Larsen-Martin, Ibid.

102 R Stewart, W Hale, "Acute Confessional States in Older Adults and the Role of Polypharmacy," *Annual Review of Health,* 13 (1992), p. 425

103 A Moraca-Sawicki, "Drug Therapy and the Older Adult," in *Pharmacotherapeutics: a Nursing Process Approach*, Ed M Kuhn (Philadelphia: F A Davis, 1998) p. 87

104 Larsen-Martin, Ibid.

105 Montamat, Cusack, "Overcoming Problems with Polypharmacy and Drug Misuse in the Elderly," *AORN Journal*, March 1999, p. 144

something that, if present, is more likely to result in an adverse health outcome.

Nurses, the health care professionals who are closest to the patients, were the first to see and report on the adverse effects of poly-pharmacy. They are also closest to the doctors who prescribe these drugs. Larsen and Martin report that the physicians willingly prescribe multiple prescriptions because they perceive (correctly) that this is what the patient wants. Little or no time is spent on the discussion of "non-prescriptive methods of treatment."

Take high blood pressure as an example. Hypertension has been called the "silent killer" because it can occur in a patient without the patient even knowing that the blood pressure is dangerously elevated. The patient may feel kind of bad, without really knowing why. When he or she meets with the physician, it is most likely the patient will be given a prescription medication that will get the blood pressure down. Many doctors prescribe beta-blockers against high blood pressure. But a new scientific study reveals that those beta-blockers prevent strokes only half as good as earlier scientific studies suggested. And more importantly, the risk for brain-infarct[106] rises. In addition, more patients get diabetes when they take beta-blockers.[107] However, high blood pressure responds quickly to a change in diet and exercise. Since this non-prescriptive method is not being used, the non-healthy life style, which was a risk factor for the disease, does not change. In fact, it is likely to get worse, and the hypertension pills become just another notch in the handle of the multi-pharmacy side-effect six-shooter.

Now, let's look at the side effects of a few of the drugs we have discussed that can result in adverse health outcomes.

Lipitor was invented by the Pfizer invention committee as a cholesterol-lowering drug. It is very profitable, making about $8 billion dollars a year. Projected profits for Lipitor for this

106 Infarct: an area of tissue that undergoes cell death due to lack of blood supply to the area

107 Der Spiegel 48/2005, p. 160

year are over $10 billion.[108] The possible side effects for this drug include fever, muscle aches, cramps, severe stomach pain, unusual tiredness, weakness, constipation, diarrhea, dizziness, gas, headache, heartburn, nausea, skin rash, minor stomach pain, birth defects, allergic reactions, "unwanted effects" in nursing babies, liver failure and, when taken "in conflict" with ten listed medications, may result in kidney failure and muscle problems.[109] There is at least one case study that suggests that Lipitor can cause severe mental problems.[110]

Plavix is used to prevent stroke and plaque buildup on artery walls. It caused adverse side effects in 13% of the test group of which there were 11,300 patients. Hemorrhaging (internal bleeding) occurred in 2% of the cases. Other side effects include neutropenia, (a deficiency of white blood cells in the blood which can lead to infection), rash and skin disorders, chest pain, accidental/inflicted injury, influenza-like symptoms, pain, fatigue, edema, hypertension, headache, dizziness, stomach pain, diarrhea, nausea, back pain, depression, coughing, bronchitis, rhinitis (a condition of sneezing, coughing, wheezing and nasal discharge) and quite a few other problems.[111] So we see the potential harm in mixing two or more of these drugs together. Does it have an adverse effect on the health of the elderly? Absolutely!

About 25% of all hospital admissions are patients who are elderly and who were admitted for adverse drug reactions caused by a multiple drug prescription. These patients come in complaining of a host of adverse side effects resulting from the multiple prescriptions of drugs; however, there have been certain patterns of adverse results that have been emerging. The medications falling into these patterns that are most often found to be associated with adverse reactions are shown here.[112]

108 JosefHasslberger,"HealthSupreme,"reportedat:http://www.newmediaexplorer.org/sepp/2004/01/31/lipitor_the_human_cost.htm

109 Drugs.Com, http://www.drugs.com/cons/lipitor.html

110 Hasslberger, Ibid.

111 Drugs.Com, Ibid.

112 Larsen-Martin, Ibid.

MEDICTIONS MOST COMMONLY ASSOCIATED WITH ADVERSE REACTIONS IN ELDERLY PATIENTS

*Psychotropic medications (particularly the benzodiazepines)
*Antihypertensive (including diuretics)
*Nonsteroidal anti-inflammatory medications
*Systemic steroids
*Theophylline
*Warfarin
*Cimetidine
*Digoxin

The number one source of trouble is *psychotropic* drugs. These are medications prescribed by psychiatrists that act on the mind. *Benzodiazepine* is a tranquilizer. "(They) can be addictive after 14 days of use. In fact, medical literature clearly cautions against prescribing tranquilizers to the elderly because of the numerous dangerous drug side effects."[113] Data from coroners' reports compiled by Britain's Home Office showed benzodiazepines as a more frequently contributing factor to causes of unnatural death each year than cocaine, heroin, ecstasy, and all other illegal drugs.[114] As the pamphlet *Elderly Abuse, Cruel Mental Health Programs,* a public service report from Citizens Commission on Human Rights states, "What is the sense of prescribing a senior citizen a tranquilizer that is more lethal and harder to withdraw from than heroin, one that leads to a 45% increase in the risk of having a car accident within seven days of taking it? Why give them an antidepressant that could increase the risk of their falling by 80%, or could cause them to become agitated or aggressive or even suicidal?"[115]

113 Tracy McVeigh, "Tranquilizers 'More Lethal Than Heroin,'" *The Observer*, 5 Nov. 2000

114 Beverly K. Eakman, "Anything That Ails You, Women on Tranqs in a Self-Serve Society," *Chronicles*, Aug. 2004

115 "Some Psychotropics May Be Inappropriate for the Elderly," *Geriatric Times,* Vol. II, Issue 2, Mar./Apr. 2001; Mort JR, Aparasu RR, "Anti-anxiety Drugs and the Elderly; For Many, Psychiatric Medications Are Inappropriately Prescribed," *Archives of Internal Medicine,* Vol.106, 2000, pp. 2825-2831

The side effects of tranquilizers are ghastly. Minor tranquilizers can cause "lethargy, lightheadedness, confusion, nervousness, sexual problems, hallucinations, nightmares, severe depression, extreme restlessness, insomnia, nausea, and muscle tremors. Epileptic seizures and death have resulted from suddenly stopping the use of minor tranquilizers."[116] And this is from the minor tranquilizers! Imagine what the major ones will do!

"Major tranquilizers, also called antipsychotics, or *neuroleptics* (nerve-seizing), frequently cause difficulty in thinking, nightmares, emotional dullness, depression, despair and sexual dysfunction. Physically, they can cause *tardive dyskinesia* -- sudden, uncontrollable, painful muscle cramps and spasms, writhing, squirming, twisting, and grimacing movements, especially of the legs, face, mouth and tongue, drawing the face into a hideous scowl."[117]

Antidepressants such as Selective Serotonin Reuptake Inhibitors can cause "headaches, nausea, anxiety and agitation, insomnia and bizarre dreams, loss of appetite, impotence and confusion."[118] As well, "it is estimated that between 10% and 25% of SSRI users experience akathisia,[119] often in conjunction with suicidal thoughts, hostility and violent behavior." As if that isn't bad enough, antidepressants can accumulate in the lungs, so that if a second antidepressant is prescribed, they may be released in toxic levels.[120]

Anti-hypertensive medications are blood-pressure reduction pills. Non-steroidal anti-inflammatory medications are those that reduce joint pain, used in the treatment of gout, arthritis and other inflammations. *Steroids*, famous for enhancing athletic

---

116 "Elderly Abuse, Cruel Mental Health Programs," *Citizens Commission on Human Rights*, 2004

117 Ibid.

118 Ibid.

119 Akathisia is a movement disorder characterized by a feeling of inner restlessness and a compulsion to be in constant motion. Often a side effect of certain drugs.

120 Reported by Japanese researchers in *The Lancet*, the Journal of the British Medical Association in 1998.

performances, are also prescribed for arthritis, kidney conditions and other uses. *Warfarin* is designed to keep blood from clotting. *Cimetidine* is used in the treatment of ulcers. *Digoxin*, for heart disease and other problems.

There is a word, "iatrogenic," which means "physician caused disease." Thus, when a doctor orders medications, or multiple medications that cause his patient to get sick, or his sickness to worsen, or results in death, the illness is considered an iatrogenic disease. In the year 2000, George Bush's Presidential Commission stated that *iatrogenic* disease was a problem of epidemic proportions. Lost income and disability costs have been estimated at close to $29 billion dollars. The number of deaths caused by these *iatrogenic* diseases is between 44,000 and 90,000 per year. It is the 8th leading cause of death among Americans. There is controversy regarding these conclusions. In the case of drug side effects, doctors would say, "Death or injury was a possible outcome. But the FDA approves the drug for use in these cases." This may be the current legal situation. But in any event, there is an undeniable accountability problem.

Drug therapy of the aged is not easy to manage. There is a possibility of causing harm. The current drug-prescribing acceptance should be challenged. There is a need to further educate health providers and patients about available non-drug therapies. Advertising should be regulated and curtailed, as it is driving the current epidemic of multiple drug prescriptions. Drug therapy should be viewed as an invasive, problem-causing technology and not as the panacea-of-all-health solutions. It is time to turn the cornucopia of drugs upside down.

THE FUTURE

What will happen to our older population when the current trend continues? When over-medication becomes the normal trend? Well, the pharmaceutical industry paints a wonderful picture. All those "Anti-Aging Movements" will talk about paradise. They are already talking about the biological ages as opposed to chronological age; they are saying that age is rising every year, that a person of 80 today feels no older than 50 of earlier years.

They talk about a lifespan of 120 and more. Anti-aging enthusiasts talk about cell research, manipulating atoms and molecules, and again and again about hormones. They talk about an allegedly GOLDEN AGE we will enter and they point to the fact that we already have 70,000 centenarians[121] in the USA that will increase to 160,000 in 2010. The fact that a *lot* of those reasons are the cause for people living longer today is not mentioned by those (paid) optimists. People live longer, in short, when they live in safe countries (no war, low criminality), when they are married, have jobs and regular work. They really live much longer when they live in the upper quarter of income (on average 4 – 6 years longer!); when they have a good education, do regular exercise and have good, healthy nutrition. In other words: a lot of the benefits of our advanced society are just *used* by the pharmaceutical PR-trumpets. They say pharmaceuticals are the cause of longevity when they are not! Even in the 18th century, medicos already knew that clean quarters and a good life with enough food contributed to the longevity of people. Today, in the so-called advanced societies, these realizations are still true.

So yes, people will live longer, we will have more centenarians, but this is *not because* the pharmaceutical industry is so busy. There are other factors for longevity, which are far more important then the newest pharmaceutical pill. But Big Pharma will continue to tell us that its sheer existence is the reason for this bright future, which is, by the way, not shared by most of the people on this planet.

We simply encounter a wrong analysis here.

Yes, there will be more and more old people tomorrow, without doubt; the demographics are right. But these old people will be bombarded with new inventions, new therapies, and new pills in the future. Old people are already a fantastic market, but Big Pharma will exploit this market even further. We will encounter advertisement statements saying it is only the matter of the right

121 Centenarians: people who are at least 100 years old

pill to live 120 years! We will encounter an optimistic television-world for the old people, which will not be true in reality for most of the elderly. Every year there will be new "inventions" and a new "magic" bullet. But behind the curtain, unseen by the most of us, there will be lots and lots of elderly people suffering from side effects. So, the more the older population consumes drugs, the more problems will appear – because every drug has side effects. Side effects will be the big issue of tomorrow. So, we will see new diseases, new misery, and new horrifying alarming news about side effects. And there will be more *iatrogenic* diseases. In the end, we will have many *drug-personalities* in the older population.

Let us hear what an expert has to say.

DR. KEVIN L. SNEAD, D.C.: "EDUCATE THE PATIENT SO HE CAN IN TURN EDUCATE OTHERS."

In today's world of the 'miracle drug,' most people, including the elderly, put their trust in their doctors for diagnosis and prescription. After all, who should better know what is wrong with the body and how to fix it? The same goes for the pharmacist. If someone has a health question, it is common to ask the local pharmacist if he has something that will handle the problem. And so it is that the patient begins by taking one medication for a body dysfunction and ends up taking more and more drugs to handle the side effects of the first one, or the next one, as far as that goes. As a result, he sometimes gets a condition that is far worse than the original illness. It is not uncommon to find patients taking many different medications at once. So what is the illogical point here? Most people do not know how their body functions, and what the drugs do to their bodies.

For this reason, one of the best ways to help a patient gain better health is to educate them on how to improve their life style so they have healthier bodies. This is what Dr. Snead firmly believes as he applies his expert chiropractic know-how on his patients. He backs up his treatments with sound education on what the body is doing and what it needs to function better. In this interview he speaks particularly about treating the old and elderly.

But first some general questions.

"What is your educational background?"

Kevin L. Snead: "I attended the Volunteer State Community College in Gallatin, Tennessee and got my Associate of Science degree in 1991. Then I went to the Regents College in New York to attain my Bachelor of Science. By 1995, I graduated from the Life University of Marietta, Georgia with a Doctor of Chiropractic Degree."

"Do you belong to any organizations?"

Kevin L. Snead: "Yes. I am currently a member of the Tennessee Chiropractic Association and also of the American Chiropractic Association. I am a member of the Better Business Bureau since 2001 and was a former member of the Georgia Chiropractic Association."

"Have you given any lectures?"

Kevin L. Snead: "I frequently do all kinds of lectures. As a matter of fact, I give a lot of them at drug-free workplaces."

"How many patients have you treated?"

Kevin L. Snead: "I have treated over 10,000 patients."

"How many of your patients were on medical drugs?"

Kevin L. Snead: "I would say that over 70% of the patients that came to me were on medical drugs."

"What were the drugs that were most commonly used?"

Kevin L. Snead: "Nowadays, many are on psychotropic drugs such as antidepressants and *Ritalin*."

"Has drug usage increased over the ten years you have been in practice?"

Kevin L. Snead: "Totally. These days people are on three to four medicines simultaneously. For example, we did some blood pressure screening for a prison recently and found that 80% of the staff members were on blood pressure medicine. The shocking thing was that they aren't on only one medication but are actually on different kinds of drugs all at the same time."

"What is your general experience with the drug increase? Are they healthier for taking the drugs? Sicker?"

Kevin L. Snead: "Well, they actually end up having more and more problems and are given more drugs to handle those new problems. Every drug has side effects. The pharmaceutical companies know this and so do the doctors. Side effects are, in most cases, written on the prescription bottle and so the patient knows them, too, but sometimes not all of the side effects are listed and so the patient and often the doctor is left in the dark. Such was the case with *Vioxx* and *Paxil*. *Vioxx* was taken off the market because, even though it handled arthritic pain, it caused heart attacks and strokes.[122] *Paxil* was found out to create violence and suicide as well as seizures, but it is still on the market today. The usual way for doctors to handle these side effects is to prescribe a medication to handle them, and, of course, these medications come with yet other side effects. It's a dwindling spiral in the long run."

"How do they justify giving patients so many drugs when the patient is just getting sicker?"

Kevin L. Snead: "It's just the fact that doctors are the opinion leaders and the pharmaceutical industry backs them up on that. People want to be healthy and they don't know how to attain it so they have to listen to what the doctor says instead of finding out what the actual problem is. Sick people act

---

122 Note: In fact, John Abramson, who wrote *Overdosed America*, (HarperCollins Publishers, 2004) states "...for every hundred people with a history of cardiovascular disease treated with Vioxx instead of naproxen there were between seven and eleven additional serious cardiovascular complications each year." Naproxen is a drug originally used to suppress the inflammation pain of arthritis.

like they have caught the physical problems when they actually acquired them. For example, people weren't born with diabetes – they acquired it. Not born with cancer – they acquired it. Not born with asthma or kidney malfunction but acquired it. Instead of figuring out why the body is breaking down and fixing it, folks end up giving it drugs. A patient will use a so-called wonder drug to take care of that symptom they are concerned about and then think if it's not hurting any more it doesn't need fixing. They go on the maxim 'if it is not broke, don't fix it,' but in this case it is not the truth. These people are just setting themselves up for more problems."

"What irritates you the most in this practice?"

Kevin L. Snead: "What gets me the worst is how people are fooled. People are so trusting in their doctors and government. They are looking through a fog. Folks just don't look at things for what and how they truly are. If they did, they would see that they would need to improve their nutrition and life style to regain health not just treat the symptoms. They would come off all those drugs and start doing something that is more effective."

"What is your pet peeve about drug usage today?"

Kevin L. Snead: "I'm particularly shocked when I look at psychiatric drugs. There are people running around totally oblivious to what is going on in their environment – like zombies. I get patients with whom I am trying to carry on a conversation, and moments later they have trouble really understanding a question about their case. Then later, I have to repeat what I went over on the first visit. They become a nuisance to themselves and to others, too, since they are not operating on all cylinders."

"Do you treat quite a few older people in your clientele today?"

Kevin L. Snead: "Yes, I do. And the problem I run into is that they are on so many different drugs that they don't even know what they are taking. It is not unusual to find them on seven – ten different medications at the same time. They have so many side effects that are treated by even more drugs, that it is hard to know what is actually happening to the first illness they began the treatment for."

"What percentage of these is of the older-age bracket?"

Kevin L. Snead: "I would say that 10 – 15% of the patients that I treat are of the older-age bracket."

"What are the drugs that older people take?"

Kevin L. Snead: "Many of them are on *Vioxx*, but they also take psychotropic drugs. The problem is that they often take so many drugs at once. Psychotropic drugs can cause serious side effects even taken alone without the addition of other drugs. Some of the elderly have dementia, and certain psychotropic drugs, such as *risperidone* (*Risperdal*), *quetiapine* (*Seroquel*), and *olanzapine* (*Zyprexa*), increase the risk of death. Taking *Valium* has shown to increase the incidence of falls causing hip fracture in the elderly. This is due to the side effects of confusion, drowsiness, and loss of muscle coordination."

"How does aging affect the use of drugs in the elderly?"

Kevin L. Snead: "With aging, a person undergoes physical changes, which affects the way medications are handled in the body. For example, the kidneys and liver no longer eliminate toxins efficiently. The heart and circulatory system aren't working at top performance anymore either. For this reason, it is easier for the elderly to overdose on the drug, and also for the body not to eliminate the drug from the body as well, meaning that the body can accumulate drugs causing an adverse effect. Side effects are increased as well. So you can imagine what seven to ten drugs being taken at once will do to the elderly."

"Are patients ever given wrong prescriptions?"

Kevin L. Snead: "Sometimes patients are given ridiculous prescriptions. For example, I once met a patient to whom a doctor wanted to prescribe *Paxil* for menstrual cramps. *Paxil* is usually prescribed for depression and panic disorder, and it does have horrible side effects. Loss of sexual drive is only one of them. Severe seizures are another. The FDA issued a warning that the drug causes suicide and violence in children under 18 years of age. However, the drug is so addictive that when the person tries to come off it, he experiences tremors, nightmares, fatigue, hallucinations, nausea, migraine headaches, mood swings and uncontrollable anger. There is even a case that happened two years ago in Wyoming when a family was awarded $6.4 million because one of their family members was on *Paxil* and killed his wife, daughter, and granddaughter. And now a doctor recommending *Paxil* for menstrual cramps? Ridiculous!"

"What side effects have you seen within your elderly drug-using patients?"

Kevin L. Snead: "I have seen one lady who had had radical mastectomy[123] done resulting in a lot of problems with pain

123 Radical mastectomy: the removal of the breast, which has been diagnosed with cancer

going into her arms and hands. She was prescribed pain pills and muscle relaxants as well as received steroid injections, but this did not result in any improvement. In fact, taking the drugs was making the condition worse, and she was tired of being sick and tired. It was only after chiropractic treatments that she started to improve. When patients are on drugs, it complicates the situation and makes it seem to the chiropractors like they are swimming up stream and not making any headway with their patients. They have to come off the drugs for any real gain to occur."

"Have you had any experience with psychotropic drug-use by the old and elderly?"

Kevin L. Snead: "This is the worst. I had a fellow in his early fifties come in who was on *Prozac* and *Lithium* – a total zombie. As well, he had received electric shock therapy and was in a terrible mess. I asked him if it helped him, and he said no. Because he was on these psychotropic drugs, he had been in a multiple car wreck. We see people on drugs like this driving on the streets and highways."

"How do you get people off of drugs?"

Kevin L. Snead: "Educating them on how the body actually works plays an important factor here. Once they see that using drugs is just asking for trouble they can decide for themselves to stop taking them. It's important to get them interested in wanting to get off the drugs, as they will then really want to do something about it. We also recommend different vitamins and minerals. A particular concoction of high dosages of vitamins and minerals, known as the 'drug bomb,' helps them with the anxiety of coming down off the drugs as well as detoxifies them. Some go to Narconon®[124]

124 Narconon®: an organization that is highly successful in the rehabilitation of alcoholics and drug addicts

and they are able to get off drugs, detoxify and replenish their minerals and vitamins quite successfully."

"What else do you tell them besides educating them?"

Kevin L. Snead: "Part of the handling is always to create a positive future for them. I tell them that taking these over-the-counter drugs is basically locking the toxins into their cells and fatty tissues. They can then see that they aren't living the healthy life style they think they are. This is important for them to come to this realization, as this will enable them to desire their own rehabilitation. There are three factors that would make their life style healthier. One is appropriate nutrition. Once off medical drugs, the vitamins and minerals are going to work in the body the way they were designed to work. The second factor is to take care of nerve interference through chiropractic treatments. And the third is to handle stress in their environment. There are different things one can do here such as self improvement courses which help a person deal with stress better."

"What vitamins and minerals do you recommend to help them with the side effects of getting off drugs?"

Kevin L. Snead: "All of them are important, but mainly, to help them handle the side effects, calcium and magnesium are of prime importance. They help with the withdrawal symptoms. Vitamins B complex and niacin are important also in that they aid in releasing toxins from the body. Calcium and magnesium also help the muscles and joints. Along with this, the patient needs to get better rest. So often, while taking these drugs, they are not sleeping very well. So this needs to be addressed as well."

"How does calcium and magnesium help with the withdrawal symptoms?"

Kevin L. Snead: "When a person has taken drugs over a period of time, they diminish the amount of minerals and calcium he has in his body, and the symptoms of this deficiency are covered up by the drugs itself. Lack of calcium causes muscle spasms, for example, especially in older people who have less calcium than the younger ones. When the person comes off drugs, this deficiency shows up in the withdrawal symptoms he now experiences. Taking magnesium diminishes the nervous reactions, and the other vitamins and minerals ease the withdrawal symptoms also."

"Have you ever experienced a case of an older person doing so much better off drugs?"

Kevin L. Snead: "Absolutely! One of my older patients was taking pills for diabetes. We got him on vitamins and minerals plus proper nutrition and got him taking exercising walks, and he no longer takes any diabetic medication. Another was on *Vioxx* for pain. He was weaned to *Ibuprofen* and after several chiropractic treatments came off all pain killer medications."

"Do chiropractic adjustments play a role in getting patients off drugs?"

Kevin L. Snead: "Indirectly it does. Chiropractic treatments help the body to relax and not be in so much pain. But the education of what the body does and what the drugs really do to the body is vitally important in getting patients off drugs. If the general population really knew what drugs and medication did, they would be very angry, and it would be very hard to sell these prescriptions to them."

"Let's go back to the subject of nutrition? There are so many theories with every day bringing a new one. What is the right one?"

Kevin L. Snead: "There is a tremendous amount of false data on dieting these days, and it is all so confusing, especially when you get so many different testimonials from different people. The important thing to do is to find out if these testimonials come from individuals who have vested interests in the company. It's the same thing with the pharmaceutical companies. They get different actors on their advertisements to speak about the new medication saying what they do to handle pain. Got pain? Do what I do. They milk it for all its worth. All this false data needs to be stripped away in order to instill the true data in the patient."

"What would you recommend as the proper nutrition for the old and elderly, and in general?"

Kevin L. Snead: "I recommend that the patient get a good multivitamin – one that is not compacted in one pill. The more that man has tinkered with the formulating of the vitamin, the less good it does for you. A general rule is if man made it, don't eat it. Unfortunately these days it's hard to get proper nutrition from our food supply. They have all kinds of preservatives and additives – all sorts of toxins to make them look good and last longer."

"What do you have to say about the drinking water these days?"

Kevin L. Snead: "The most important thing is to drink a lot of good water and not the filtered water or cleaned with reverse osmosis[125]. That is just junk. And tap water is

125 Reverse osmosis: a process used to purify the drinking water

totally junk. Even when they say they clean up the water, it is definitely not clean. It has all that chlorine in it that clogs our arteries causing heart problems in the end for the older population. That is not clean. Even when dairy products are homogenized and pasteurized, it clogs arteries, but drinking water is the real point here. A person with a 200-cholesterol count can die of artery blockage, whereas another guy who has 400-cholesterol count and who does not have the proper nutrition, doesn't have a heart attack because he drinks reverse osmosis drinking water. It's a falsity that the cholesterol gives you a heart attack. It doesn't. If one has scarred arteries and 100-cholesterol count, the arteries are going to clog. What I instill in my patients is that the best bet is to drink spring water – something that hasn't had anything added to it. I also recommend calcium and magnesium."

"How about eating meat?"

Kevin L. Snead: "I don't think there is a problem with eating meat. Probably better to eat duck than pork, but I don't insist upon what people eat. I do recommend that the patient lay off of the sugar and eat lots of vegetables. Raw would be good. But even the vegetables aren't really that good today as they were when our parents were around. The soil is so depleted. It is best to stay with organic food – food that hasn't been treated with herbicides and pesticides and other chemicals to make them look good and last longer."

"What causes the soil to be so depleted?"

Kevin L. Snead: "Well for one thing the modern agricultural practices are at fault here. There is intensive farming with poor crop rotation as well as chemical re-fertilization and genetic modification. Pesticides are so widely used that there is even documented evidence that popular foods are being contaminated. So we have toxic residues along with our vegetables. Even the fruit along with the vegetables have often been in cold storage for six to nine months and this will cause the nutrient content to decrease drastically. That's why a good vitamin and mineral supplement is necessary."

"Is there a special diet for older people?"

Kevin L. Snead: "I don't put older people on special diets. I recommend a balanced diet along with a good vitamin and mineral supplement. It's important that they get enough protein and not just loading up on sugar and carbohydrates. As for carbohydrates there are better carbohydrates and sugar carbohydrates. I suggest they go for the better carbohydrates."

"What would you say are the better carbohydrates?"

Kevin L. Snead: "Actually carbohydrates are separated into simple carbohydrates and complex carbohydrates. The simple carbohydrates contain sugar and few vitamins and minerals. They include such foods as yogurt, molasses, sugar, and milk and are digested quickly into the body. The complex carbohydrates would be a better choice. These are foods that take longer to digest such as vegetables, cereals, and legumes."

"What about processed foods?"

Kevin L. Snead: "It is always better to avoid refined foods that are high in sugar. And also better to eat food that is closer to its natural form. Foods that are refined have been handled a lot, and each time you do something else with that food you get fewer nutrients. Exposure to heat and air, or otherwise altering it, destroys the nutrients in the food. For example, bagged, peeled vegetables and fruits or bagged cut lettuce and salad blends have exposed the vegetable or fruit to the air and there is significant vitamin and mineral loss when you do that. Even eating a whole apple is better that eating the apple sauce since the heat and air exposure destroys the nutrients."

"What is the difference between diets of elderly people and younger people?"

Kevin L. Snead: "There is definitely a big difference. Today's children are grown up on MacDonald's and all the other fast food while the elderly people are still eating lots of vegetables and arresting their intake of meat."

"In theory, should elderly people elect a special nutrition in relation to the younger generation?"

Kevin L. Snead: "As you get older a lot of systems wear out especially when folks are on so many different medications. The body also does not assimilate most of the foods the way it was when it was 30 to 40 years old. This should be taken into account."

"What is your special motto for the business you are in?"

Kevin L. Snead: "Educate the patient so he can, in turn, educate others."

4. DANGER! WHAT DRUGS ARE DOING TO OUR CHILDREN

There is more than one scandal when it comes to the subject "children and drugs." The biggest one we will save for the end of this chapter. But if one truly wants to understand the intentions of the pharmaceutical drug cartel in relation to our children, one must look at some *data* first. So let's examine some objective information.

In 2000, 70.4 million children under the age of 18 lived in the United States. The number of children under 18 has nearly doubled since 1950. In 2010, we will have about 72 million children in the USA, and by the year 2020, 77.2 million, says the *USA Census Bureau.* We will face many more Hispanic children in the future, a few more black children, and about the same amount of white children.

However, we are talking about 72 million children here. Now let us take, for a moment, the viewpoint of a mother who has to raise a child. Usually mothers are responsible for the kids, despite the fact that mothers today generally have to work. In the good old times, mothers could just stay at home, which was probably better for raising children. So what is a mother up against, today?

KIDS AND SICKNESS

Most mothers would agree that the best sound in the world is that of her child's laughter. It simply infuses her with joy. On the flip side, the worst sound, one that sends shivering shards of anxiety up and down her spine, is the sound of her child in pain. A good parent would do anything, absolutely anything to spare their child from hurt. The question, when a child is sick, is what is the best long-term remedy? How does a mother protect her child from pain?

One of the first things a new parent realizes is that there are hundreds of decisions to make, seemingly, on a daily basis. Most of them are extremely important and have advocates with polar viewpoints making life seem like a field of land mines. One of the first decisions will be to vaccinate or not to vaccinate? Type the question into your favorite search engine on the Internet and you will discover a war on the subject. Is the climbing rate of autism in the United States linked to all the vaccinations children receive? Ask 20 friends if they have known anyone who was adversely affected by vaccinations and the result will be a surprise.

Okay, next scenario. It is 2 AM and little six-month-old baby Sam wakes up screaming in pain. Mama rushes to his side and discovers that he is warm to the touch. Panicked, she calls her pediatrician who advises mama to give the child a pain killer/ fever suppressant and to call her office in the morning to set an appointment. Relieved to have a solution, mama gives her baby son *Tylenol* and puts him back in his crib. Somewhere in the back of her mind, she knows that a body's natural defense to an illness is to raise its temperature, but mama can't think straight when her child is crying, so she blindly follows the advice of the pediatrician.

The next morning she visits the doctor, who checks the baby's ears, finds them red and prescribes an antibiotic. Perhaps, mama has read up on the overuse of antibiotics and the hazards of giving them to a child willy-nilly. If she's lucky, her pediatrician will admit that she doesn't know what is causing the earache. The educated doctor will advise her to wait and see if the infection improves on its own. She would prescribe pain-relieving eardrops instead and schedule the baby for a follow up visit in a couple of days.

If mama isn't so lucky, the pediatrician will insist on the antibiotic and an unfortunate pattern has begun. For one thing, the earache may or may not be improved by the antibiotic. If it was a virus and not a bacterial infection, the antibiotic will have no effect, except to wipe out the good bacteria in the system and possibly promote allergies later in life.

Another problem is that the bacteria that cause certain ear infections are becoming increasingly resistant to antibiotics. What is the medical solution? Prescribe a higher dose of antibiotic.

According to Dr. Allan Greene, the problem is that "each time a child takes a course of antibiotics, future infections become harder to treat." In addition, he reports, "Of the 10 million annual antibiotic prescriptions for ear infections, somewhere between 8.5 million and 9.5 million prescriptions didn't actually help the children."[126]

There are a number of homeopathic and naturopathic remedies that have been successful, and often simply waiting out the earache will take care of the problem. Of course the best way to prevent illness is to ensure our children eat the best organic foods and are breastfed as long as possible.

Now, let's fast-forward a decade. Baby Sam is now 10 years old and he is on a typical American diet of sugar, carbohydrates and television. His teacher calls mama in for a parent/teacher conference, because her child is not concentrating well in class. Teacher also has noticed that the child gets depressed sometimes and is "overly active" at other times. She strongly suggests that mama take the child to a psychiatrist. Again, mama is reading up on the latest information about parenting and is hesitant to take her son to a psychiatrist, knowing that about eight million children are currently taking anti-depressant drugs. Not wanting to risk that battle, she politely declines the teacher's request.

If she is lucky, the teacher will not insist. If she is unlucky, the school might threaten to remove the child from her custody should she refuse a psychiatric evaluation. Now, mama may be forced to give her child a powerful mind-altering drug, which has a host of side effects including nausea, involuntary twitching, insomnia, painful muscle cramping and many other problems.

The child's depression may simply be an allergic reaction to some food he ate, a sugar low from the Frosted Flakes he had for breakfast or perhaps he is just deficient in certain minerals or vitamins. Or it could be possible he is just a normal child fighting the average ups and downs of being a pre-teen.

By the time Sam has become an adult, he has probably had a complete set of vaccinations, dozens (if not hundreds) of rounds of

---

126 Dr. Allan Greene, "A Welcome Revolution in Ear Infection Treatment," March 11, 2002 and http://www.drgreene.com/21_1771.html

antibiotics, various painkillers, anesthetics and perhaps some anti-depressants. His body no longer works properly, and he finds that he catches every single common cold and flu that goes around the office routinely.

ANTIBIOTICS

Now, let us change back to a more objective viewpoint. At least, one should have some sort of an opinion on vaccinations, antibiotics and psychotropic drugs – drugs that affect the mental health of the child.

Let us take up the controversial subject of antibiotics first. What are usually not known about antibiotics are its side effects. The repeated course and overuse of antibiotics can end in chronic fatigue syndrome, diabetes, and even cancer.[127] Antibiotics, once the talk of the day, a medication which saved many lives and which is useful in killing some deadly bacteria infections, is today overused by many doctors. The medical doctor has to prescribe something and so he prescribes what? Yes, antibiotics. They don't help in the case of virus infections and in some of the chronic diseases. Some critics estimate that at least more then *half* of all antibiotic prescriptions are unnecessary, including antibiotics given to children; other critics say 90% are useless. (i.e. the author Erica Heilmann) In hospitals, antibiotics are given on a routine basis – "just in case." Especially for children, the side effects can be horrifying. *The British National Formulary* reveals, "Prolonged use of the antibiotic *neomycin*[128] to treat liver diseases can cause the liver to malfunction. *Tetracycline* can permanently stain a child's teeth yellow, the antibiotic chloramphenicol[129] can interfere with the bone marrows production

127 Lyyne McTaggart, Ibid. p. 181

128 *Neomycin* is mainly used topically in the treatment of skin and mucous membrane infections, wounds, and burns. Although it is also used systemically, it is highly toxic. http://reference.allrefer.com/encyclopedia/N/neomycin.html

129 *Chloramphenicol* is used in the treatment of infections caused by bacteria. It works by killing bacteria or preventing their growth. http://health.yahoo.com/health/drug/202127/

of red blood cells and cause irreversible, potentially fatal, bone-marrow depression."[130] "General overuse of antibiotics can damage the immune-system, cause gastrointestinal disorders, and lead to allergies, psoriasis and even multiple sclerosis."[131] One could go and on and quote the literature, but the point is: even an originally "good" drug, a medication which definitely has its use from time to time, one of the great inventions of modern medicine, is overused and inappropriately used on a routine basis today. The authors guess that the side effects of antibiotics today far exceed the plus side of this medication. (A good book to read on this subject is *The Killers Within, The Deadly Rise of Drug-resistant Bacteria* by Michael Shnayerson and Mark J. Plotkin.)

So let us look at the FACTS at a glance:

FACT: Antibiotics don't work for viral infections.

FACT: Half of all antibiotics, up to 90% of all antibiotics administered/prescribed, are unnecessary.

FACT: The overuse of antibiotics can cause bacteria to mutate so that antibiotics no longer work in the end. The more antibiotics you use, the more drug resistance you see.

FACT: If you overuse antibiotics, it is possible you will run out of treatment options. Even for bacterial infections, which are still treatable at the moment.

FACT: (Mild) Adverse reactions to antibiotics: Yeast infections, stomach upset.

FACT: (Heavy) Adverse reactions to antibiotics: allergic reactions, chronic fatigue syndrome, diabetes, cancer.

Any more questions?

---

130 Lynne McTaggart, p. 190

131 Lynne McTaggart, p. 191

VACCINATIONS

History taught us how important vaccinations are. Nevertheless, there is hardly any other subject which is, meanwhile, as controversial as the subject of vaccination.

Past generations thought vaccination successful: 1878, smallpox defeated; 1885, rabies; 1911, typhoid; 1921, tuberculosis; 1925, diphtheria and tetanus; 1937, yellow fever; 1954, polio; 1960, measles; and 1967, mumps.

Today, every child in the USA is vaccinated against whooping cough, hepatitis, chickenpox, measles, polio, diphtheria, mumps and tetanus. In fact there are 40 recommended childhood immunizations in all as of January 2002. If parents resist, they come into conflict with the law. Vaccinations, so it seems, are the great unquestionable victory of modern medicine. And it is true: millions of lives have been saved because of vaccinations. Louis Pasteur, Robert Koch, Emil von Behring and many other researchers *are* heroes.

The only thing wrong with vaccinations is that there are new scientific findings, which indicate that vaccinations can be a great danger as well. The amount of vaccinations people take today is especially startling, because every vaccination has it side effects. Researcher Harris L. Coulter estimates that 1000 babies, at a minimum, die from DPT, (diphtheria-pertussis-tetanus vaccination) every year, while 12,000 are permanently damaged.[132] And how about Sudden Infant Death Syndrome?[133] This is often linked with vaccination reactions. Ten thousand American babies mysteriously die each year from this catchall disease.[134]

The medical establishment sings the song of silence when it comes to those side effects.

---

132 Harris L. Coulter, *Vaccination, Social Violence, and Criminality*, (North Atlantic Books, California 1990)

133 Sudden Infant Death Syndrome: also known as crib death, a fatal syndrome that affects sleeping infants under a year old, wherein the baby suddenly stops breathing

134 Tim O'Shea, *The Sanctity of Human Blood, Vaccination is not Immunization*, (North Woods, 2003), p. 54

Here is just one more example. The side effects following smallpox vaccination can cause severe skin infections, sometimes destroying tissue and causing permanent disability. Or vaccine can even affect the eyes and permanently cause blindness.[135]

Other authors cite cases suggesting a link between MMR (Mumps-Measles-Rubella-vaccination) and autism.[136] Other warns: "Half of the American population suffers from skin allergies, allergic rhinitis,[137] bronchial asthma of allergic origin, food allergies, and other. The prevalence of allergies is steadily rising in all industrial societies. This creeping epidemic could well be one more long-term effect on our increasingly widespread and all-encompassing childhood vaccination programs."[138]

Critic Harris L. Coulter states that vaccinations can cause neurological disabilities and so could be the real source for the increase in criminality. Coulter considers further the relationship of vaccination to autism, hyperactivity, autoimmune diseases and learning disabilities.

Well, here are the facts: Childhood vaccinations *can* cause various types of mental retardation ranging from a slight drop in IQ to total idiocy. Meanwhile, 9% of the people in the USA during the years 1946 to 1966 are illiterates, the *Census Bureau* tells us. Mere chance?

Another fact: "Today, about 3,000,000 children are born every year in the United States. Of them, 150,000 develop less severe handicaps; 110,000 more severe ones."[139]

And there is more: 31% of United States children suffer from a chronic condition. Again, mere chance? We don't think so. As Dr. Mendelsohn wrote over 15 years ago, "There is a growing suspicion that immunization against harmless childhood diseases

---

135 Lawrence K. Altman, "Smallpox Proposal Raises Ethical Issue," *The New York Times*, June 22, 2002

136 Andrew Wakefield and Associates, *The Lancet*, British Medical Journal, 1998

137 Rhinitis: Inflammation of the mucous membrane of the nose

138 Coulter, p. 151

139 Coulter, p. 258

may be responsible for the dramatic increase in autoimmune diseases since mass inoculations were introduced… ……cancer, leukemia, rheumatoid arthritis, MS, Lou Gehrig's disease, lupus, and Guillain-Barre' syndrome."[140] It is no wonder then that quite a few health-professionals *warn* us about the repercussions of vaccinations. They propose a minimum of vaccinations. They propose more intense research in relation to long-term side effects, and propose not to inoculate babies, the very young.

THE HIDDEN AGENDA

But what is the agenda behind all this countless number of vaccinations? Well, vaccinations will increase in our opinion for two reasons:

1. The biological warfare causes panic.
2. Vaccinations are a huge income source.

And now it becomes extremely exciting. Just look. Billions of dollars were just recently spent on the recent wars (Afghanistan, Iraq). We very quickly see that one can make a lot of money with terror-threats. Yes, most of the money was spent in the direction of the weapon-dealers, the weapon-construction companies; but a huge portion also went to Big Pharma.

Just one single bit of information comes to the forefront: in June 2002, President George W. Bush signed into law a $4.6 billion bio-terrorism prevention program, of which $640 million went to the production and stockpile of smallpox-vaccine.[141] We don't have to be deep-thinking philosophers to see the future. Of course, *more* money will be spent on potential biological warfare, and there will be one winner: the Pharmaceutical industry.

Aside from the political situation, vaccinations are, in any case, an unbelievable cash cow. Vaccinations, despite some horrible side effects and possibly even more disastrous long-term side effects, *always* mean a lot of money, war or no war. When entire populations

140 Mendelsohn, M.D., *How to Raise a Healthy Child In Spite Of Your Doctor,* (Ballantine, New York, 1984), p. 165

141 See Gary Null, ibid. p. 126

have to be inoculated against some disease, imagine that! – That is the real deal.

Vaccine production is big business. The pharmaceutical giant Merck, for example, rakes in $900 million every year. Since vaccinations still have an excellent image, it is easy to convince people to be inoculated. Billions of dollars are earned here. But guess who pays for those afflicted with adverse reactions? The taxpayer. And yet, new vaccinations are continuously researched and tested for; many are underway at this very moment as these lines are written.

The authors of this book believe that the true danger of mass-vaccinations is not realized. So here are some more facts:

FACT: Critics suggest that many more cases of death occur as a result of vaccination than officially reported. Less than 10% of actual ill effects are reported. In fact, there was no reporting agency in place before 1991, so no one knows how many died or suffered from adverse reactions before then.[142] And to top that off there are no follow-ups of the reports. None!

FACT: The incidences of serious adverse reactions are unquestionable, which may be in the order of magnitude of hundreds of thousands every year in the USA. Some authors (like Canadian author Guylaine Lanctot, MD., who wrote the bestseller *Medical Mafia*) conclude that medical authorities are not telling the truth about the actual side effects of vaccinations.[143]

FACT: Vaccinations, on the other hand, can sometimes cause an outbreak of the actual inoculated disease later.

FACT: Vaccinations can suppress the immune systems and make the person weaker to other diseases.

---

142 Tim O'Shea, *The Sanctity of Human Blood, Vaccination is not Immunization,* (North Woods, 2003), p. 62

143 See http://www.med-library.net/content/view/319/41/

FACT: Flue vaccine often does not work on an amazing amount of people. Yet health officials promote flu vaccinations.[144]

FACT: Vaccinations can cause bacteria and viruses to mutate to become resistant. Then, later, those bacteria are even more dangerous. Does the pharmaceutical industry create the new diseases of tomorrow?

In a way, we face here the same problem as with antibiotics. Originally a great invention, the overuse of vaccinations can lead to deadly consequences. Since the whole nation is educated into the blind belief that vaccinations are great, the whole population is at risk. What will happen when this trend continues? Here's a possible scenario.

FUTURE: Some madmen could mutate bacteria so that biological warfare will be possible even for a small amount of people. Even billions of dollars will not protect us.

FUTURE: The people who "help" in respect to a possible biological warfare are just those people who created the weapons in the first place, health officials, because they breed bacteria. Imagine they get stolen, or, in the case of Russia, sold to madmen. Especially genetically engineered bacteria can become resistant.

FUTURE: Under a crazy government (influenced by Big Pharma), it could very well be that, under a bioterrorism attack, the entire population is forced to receive vaccinations and suffer horrible side effects.

FUTURE: How would the pharmaceutical industry sell those mass-vaccinations?

144 Informed consent advocate says government and industry should release flu vaccine effectiveness data. http://www.vaccineinfo.net/immunization/vaccine/influenza/flu_vaccine_facts.shtml: "The flu vaccine only protects against the three specific viral strains which are included in any given year's flu vaccine. Throat, respiratory, gastrointestinal and ear infections caused by bacteria or other kinds of viruses are not prevented by getting an annual flu shot."

Via the government of course by their own lobby, the media that concentrates in selling fear. And via *front groups*. Front groups that are *not* grass-root movements. Artificial front groups. False front-groups are a piece of technology of the black propaganda know-how. We will talk more about that later.

Do we know what is really on the hidden agenda of the pharmaceutical drug cartel?

It is interesting to note, at this point, that the concerns of drugging children and the side effects created by the drugs have been brought up by the Psychopharmacologic Drugs Advisory Committee and the Pediatric Subcommittee of the Anti-infective Drugs Advisory Committee. At a meeting in February 2004, they discussed the "… concerns about reports of suicidal ideas and behavior developing in some children and adolescents during treatment of depression with an SSRI[145] or similar newer antidepressant."[146] So you see that they are not blind to this fact. It was even stated, "… major depression among thousands of the nation's youth was under-diagnosed, understudied, and under-treated."[147]

And yet with this in mind, they are still prescribing drugs as if children were laboratory guinea pigs, without really doing the full research needed to warrant the use of these drugs. Horrifying! We will take up this scandal in a moment, but first let's take a look at what else came up in that meeting.

Dr. Kratz, the Division Director of the Division of Neuropharmacological Drug Products, FDA, stated that the drug Paxil was recommended to not be used to treat pediatric patients.[148]

145 SSRI: (selective serotonin reuptake inhibitor) a class of drugs, such as fluoxetine or sertraline, that inhibit the uptake of serotonin by neurons of the central nervous system and are primarily used in the treatment of depression and obsessive compulsive disorder.

146 Minutes of the meeting convened by the Department of Health and Human Services Food and Drug Administration Center for Drug Evaluation and Research held on February 2, 2004. http://www.fda.gov/ohrms/dockets/ac/04/transcripts/4006T1.htm pp. 12 – 13

147 http://www.fda.gov/ohrms/dockets/ac/04/transcripts/4006T1.htm p. 14

148 http://www.fda.gov/ohrms/dockets/ac/04/transcripts/4006T1.htm p. 21

PSYCHIATRIC DRUGS

Now we come to the scandal of all scandals: *psychotropic* drugs.

Psychotropic simply means drugs, which affect a person's mental state, his psyche – a big word for a non-complicated thing. *Tropic* means simply 'affecting.' Since Big Pharma found out that children are a fantastic market, every effort has been undertaken to put children on drugs. The scandal is not even the fact that Big Pharma tried to take the decision of children using psychotropic drugs or not out of the hand of parents and into the hands of public school administrators, so that suddenly, parents potentially no longer had any right to determine if their own child had to take a psychotropic drug or not.[149] No, the real scandal is that children are degraded to a *market.* They are used for money. Children cannot yet think for themselves. They are turned into drug-personalities without knowing it. Children are educated into being drug-takers, drug consumers from the earliest childhood on.

But how did Big Pharma "develop" this target-market?

Well, with the invention of new diseases of course. Aaaah, we instantly had two wonderful "disorders" children could be diagnosed with. Wonderful! Today one just says that a child has *ADD* or *ADHD*. What does that mean? Well *ADD* means *Attention Deficit Disorder*, a big term meaning nothing more than the child cannot keep his attention long enough on a subject. *ADHD* just means *Attention Deficit Hyperactivity Disorder*, which just adds hyperactivity to the inability to focus attention. Now the scandal here is that this can be "diagnosed" by observation alone, NOT by an objective scientific test. Who knows what the real source for the child's attention-deficit is? The psychiatrists say that it is caused by a chemical imbalance. But the American Psychiatric Association President, Steven Sharfstein,

149 In 2003, the USA New Freedom Commission on Mental Health recommended, as influenced by psychiatrists and psychologists, that there be "...early detection of mental health problems in children and adults – through routine and comprehensive testing and screening." – "Harming Youth, Psychiatry Destroys Young Minds," *CCHR*, 2004.

admitted on the TODAY show that there is no way to test for a "chemical imbalance" as the cause for mental disorders.[150] He said, "We do not have a clean-cut lab test."[151] Thus, it may NOT AT ALL be caused by a chemical reason, the parents might be troublesome at home, the dog may have died, or the dolls not have the right clothes. You understand? Very arbitrary. One can "diagnose" a child as "sick" with a new expression, a chic expression.

But let us be a bit more "scientific," despite the fact there hardly exists any term that is more misused than the word "science." Over 134,000,000 prescriptions of *psychotropic* drugs in the USA were dispensed in 2004 alone. "Six million kids are on Ritalin daily." Currently in the USA, over 4000 kids are put onto *Prozac* for the first time. PER DAY. Twelve thousand seven hundred and thirty-one gallons of liquid Prozac have been handed out in the public school system in Los Angeles within 3 months in 2004. This all happened because children were diagnosed with ADHD *(Attention Deficit Hyperactivity Disorder)*. Now again, the bad joke is the fact that there isn't a 100% diagnosis for this "disease." Just read one description:

ADHD predominantly inattentive type: (ADHD-I)5

- *Fails to give close attention to details or makes careless mistakes.*
- *Has difficulty sustaining attention.*
- *Does not appear to listen.*
- *Struggles to follow through on instructions.*
- *Has difficulty with organization.*
- *Avoids or dislikes tasks requiring sustained mental effort.*
- *Loses things.*
- *Is easily distracted.*
- *Is forgetful in daily activities.*[152]

150 TODAY Show interview (27 June)

151 *PEOPLE Magazine*, (11July)

152 http://www.chadd.org/fs/fsl.htm

ADHD predominately hyperactive-impulsive type: (ADHD-HI)5

- *Fidgets with hands or feet or squirms in chair.*
- *Has difficulty remaining seated.*
- *Runs about or climbs excessively.*
- *Difficulty engaging in activities quietly.*
- *Acts as if driven by a motor.*
- *Talks excessively.*
- *Blurts out answers before questions have been completed.*
- *Difficulty waiting or taking turns.*
- *Interrupts or intrudes upon others.*[153]

Do you understand how questionable those criteria are? There is plenty of room for interpretation. A doctor can label any child very easy with a "disease" this way. At the same time, those "experts" state: "Nonetheless, the exact causes of ADHD remain illusive" and: ".... A diagnostic test for ADHD does not exist." So imagine: no single test is in existence for this disorder. There are theories of "comprehensive evaluations," but let us repeat "no single test is in existence." There is a host of diagnostic problems. Nevertheless, this "disease" gets diagnosed over and over.

The first diagnostic mistake is the fact that there may be many different reasons for a child to be hyperactive or be unable to focus. Sugar, an incorrect diet, problems at home, being on drugs or alcohol, lack of vitamins or minerals, Candida, yeast, spinal subluxations,[154] to name a few, can contribute to this condition. Of course, the pharmaceutical drug cartel fights all those very obvious reasons. But it is a plain fact, on the other hand, that this "disease" isn't necessarily a chemically caused problem. So the diagnostic problem is a dilemma. However, one thing we know for sure. The drugs, which allegedly fight this disorder, *do* have side effects, from fatigue to passivity, from fear to depression. What then? Then the "experts" use stimulant medications. And what do they do when

153 ibid.

154 Subluxations: a partial dislocation of a bone in a joint

drug addiction is the result? Right. They try to invent a drug to cure drug addiction, not seeing that the *cure* is the *disease.*

Again: ADHD means *Attention Deficit Hyperactivity Disorder.* Wonderful, wonderful term that sounds so intelligent, so scientific and it is the biggest fraud one can imagine! We, the authors, think that a huge activity, as long as it points in constructive directions, is a *good* sign – an excellent sign indeed. It shows the child is healthy and *alive*. Well yes, some may not like it, some "George Orwell *1984*" fanatics want a society that is obedient, silent, calm and doesn't make trouble. But WHO, for God's sake, says that this is "normal"? It could very well be that the revolutionary attitude is the sane attitude. People who were able to disagree, who were obsessed by an idea, who were "hyperactive," who worked night and day, have caused a lot of big changes in our society, leading us into a better world. With this new kind of philosophy, we are moving into a world of obedience, of mental slavery, of obsessive adaptation and conformity. Yes, it is practical and makes less work when a child isn't "hyperactive." But perhaps we destroy our children when we define (and agree) to a standard that is stopping our children, which is scientifically questionable and, in the final end, opinion and nothing more than opinion.

But we don't even have to be that complicated in arguing; the real truth is much simpler. With a "hyperactive" child Big Pharma can make *money*. Big Pharma (with the help of some mind-healers) just created a new arbitrary definition of mental "illness" and mental "health" and can fill its pockets.

In a heartbeat, we have a new "risk-factor" – fantastic! *Hyperactivity.* We have a new market, and now billions of dollars more can be earned. So simple is the real truth. The long and the short of it is that an insane hyperactivity (hyperactivity that is destructive, as opposed to an increased activity which is towards creativity) may be very well traced to other sources. The true source for hyperactive is NOT handled by drugs, but, perhaps, by good control through good communication to children from the adults in their environment. To reduce hyperactivity to brain-chemistry, how primitive can this judgment be? But again, the simpler truth is: here we have a wonderful *market.*

Nothing against the billions of dollars earned with a new definition, a new risk factor, and a new disease. Only an intellectual PR-genius can make those billions. So nothing against it … if …, if …, yes if there wouldn't be those horrible side effects.

The side effects of *Ritalin,*[155] *Metadate CD,*[156] and *Adderall?*[157]

What are the possible side effects? Well a*ddiction* is only one possible scenario. But the fact is teenagers taking psychotropic drugs have committed more than half of the last 12 school shootings. *Ritalin,* the most commonly prescribed psychiatric drug for children, is currently administrated to one in every 30 children between the ages of 5 and 18, but *Ritalin* is classified in the same group of drugs as opium, morphine and cocaine. Side effects of its use include: *stunted growth, weight loss, maniac behavior, future drug dependence, heart palpitations, cardiac arrhythmia, anxiety, insomnia, violent behavior and even death.*[158]

Violence is one result of this, *anxiety* another. *Maniac behavior* (artificially enthusiastic and crazy about something) and body sicknesses, including *death*, may be the case.

Currently, there is something called TeenScreen. The plan of psychiatry is to do regular check-ups of children in schools, health care facilities, juvenile justice and child welfare organizations.[159] Screening is done without actual medical tests but by survey alone of the child to see if he or she is suicidal. Depending on the answers

155 *Ritalin* is a mild stimulant to the central nervous system (brain and nerves). The exact way that Ritalin works is unknown.

156 *Methylphenidate* is a mild stimulant to the central nervous system (brain and nerves). The exact way that methylphenidate works is unknown.

157 *Adderal* is a stimulant and appetite suppressant. It stimulates the central nervous system (nerves and brain) by increasing the amount of certain chemicals in the body. This increases heart rate and blood pressure and decreases appetite, among other effects.

158 Karen Hadley, "Singer Appeals to DCs for the Children," *The Chiropractic Journal*: August 2004

159 *The Communication Line*, 19 April 2005, p. 2

given, the teen is then put on mentally damaging drugs. What is ironic is that the psychiatrists have the highest rate of suicide (about 5 times) amid their ranks as compared to the general population. Who are they then to diagnose suicidal tendency? The questions alone are ambiguous (example: has there been a time when you felt you couldn't do anything well?) and are easily answered "yes." Again the drugs prescribed may be creating the suicide rather than handling it.[160]

Just recently, a study was completed, documenting that 96 Florida children ages 18 and under committed suicide after using psychotropic drugs. This is over a five-year period from 1999 to 2004 and represents 38% of the total youth suicides. Florida State Representative, Gus Barreiro, released the report February 23, 2006, which also showed that 36 children who had committed suicide were using the popular *ADHD* stimulant medications, which are given to some 2.5 million children in America today. Barreiro stated, "These drugs are dangerous and there is no question that they kill children. Parents need to know the consequences. We fully expect this bill to pass through the legislature this year and we hope that the Governor will sign it into law. It is long past due."[161]

Drugs for Attention Deficit Disorder (ADD) may also cause *permanent changes* to the brains of children taking them.

Movements that protest these psychotropic drugs have already come into existence. The protesters point out the fact that many famous people, according to modern "science," would have been diagnosed with "Attention Deficit Disorder" or "Hyperactivity" – lots of creative people in fact. So someone who is different, not fitting into the norm, into the box, is "sick" like Bill Crosby, Dustin Hoffman, James Stewart, Kirk Douglas, Robin Williams, Sylvester Stallone? Harry Belafonte, Cher, Pablo Picasso, Edgar Allan Poe, Ernest Hemingway, Bernhard Shaw, Jules Verne and Agatha Christie had ADD?[162]

---

160 Elyse Van Breemen, "Say NO To Mental Health Screening Of Teens," *The Communication Line*, 22 November 2005, pp 1 – 2

161 http://hanseisenman.typepad.com/health/2006/02/suicidal_teens_.html#more

162 http://www.oneaddplace.com/famous.htm

We don't think so. But nevertheless, this is fact: eight million children a year, which is about 10% of the school-aged population, are prescribed behavior-changing and mind-altering drugs today for "learning and attention difficulties." Today there are 17 million children worldwide consuming mind-altering drugs.[163] And psychotropic drugs are just the tip of the iceberg. We haven't even mentioned the increasing number of teens using prescription drugs, particularly painkillers, every day. "*The National Institute on Drug Abuses*" reported that 10.5% of 12th graders use *Vicodin*[164] for non-medical reasons and 4.5% of 12th graders reported are using *OxyContin*[165] without prescription.

We didn't mention children's aspirin, which can cause Reye's syndrome, an illness with inflammation of brain, fever, vomiting, and progressive coma.

We didn't mention the FDA approved drug *Depentum* (for adults only), but the drug company claimed it is safe for children too.

We didn't mention all the brand names of existing stimulants, antidepressants, anti-anxiety medications, anti-psychotic-medications and other medications our children are fed today.

We didn't mention, "two thirds of all drugs they [pediatricians] routinely prescribe have never been adequately studied on kids, according to a study by Food and Drug Administration researchers."[166]

We didn't quote examples, such as the case of some drugs (chloramphenicol, an antibiotic) normally used on adults, being used on newborn babies who died after receiving this drug.[167]

163 "Harming Youth, Psychiatry Destroys Young Minds," *Citizens Commission on Human Rights*, 2004

164 *Vicodin* is indicated for the relief of moderate to moderately severe pain.

165 *OxyContin* is in a class of drugs called narcotic analgesics. It is a pain reliever.

166 http://www.boston.com/yourlife/health/children/articles/2003/08/20/most_drugs_never_tested_for_safety_in_children/

167 http://pubs.acs.org/subscribe/journals/mdd/v07/i03/pdf/304rules.pdf

We didn't talk about the under-dosing, overdosing and ineffectiveness of many drugs given to our children.

We didn't bring up the fact that, today, more and more children are being put on drugs; of course the pharmaceutical industry calls it "better drugs." Why? Because it would distract us from the true scandal which is again: *Children are looked at as a market.* Big Pharma leads our children, our teens in the direction of addiction. Why? For money! Children are a "wonderful" market, because we care so much for our children.

NEW MARKETS

So to summarize:

The use of medication for children is on the rise. Asthma, behavior problems, colds, infections, diabetes, depression, all those "diseases" are treated today with heavy drugs. On the other hand, the side effects are fantastic. More and more children take medications to treat depression, ADHD, and behavioral conditions; they are treated with *Prozac*[168] or *Zoloft.*[169] Despite the fact that the pharmaceutical drug cartel makes money. And the psychiatric profession helps.

Wonderful, wonderful markets!

Bedwetting and specific fears are treatable. The little ones have so many fears – isn't that great? School phobia, separation anxiety, fear of leaving home, sadness, helplessness, hopelessness, guilt, eating disorder, maniac-depressive condition (periods of depression alternative with happy moods, excessive energy, staying up late at night, grand plans, etc), strange behavior, extreme stubbornness, persistent rituals, irrational belief – all that can be treated. Allegedly!

Drugs, drugs, drugs. Oh, we have wonderful, stimulate medications such as *Ritalin*; and we have anti-depressants,

168 *Prozac* is documented with having caused suicide in quite a few cases.

169 *Zoloft* is a drug used in the treatment of depression, panic disorder, obsessive-compulsive disorder, and post-traumatic stress disorder.

antipsychotic drugs, tranquilizers such as *Haldol,*[170] and *Lithium*[171] for the manic-depressives (now called Bipolar disorder). In fact, one could invent or name at least 101 more anxieties. All those anxieties can become future markets one day. Markets, markets, markets.

One really must restrain oneself not to be cynical here, but we are far away from cynicism. All those "disorders" and "diseases" *are* already treated – with partially horrible side effects.

THE FUTURE

Imagine that there are more and more children and teens taking drugs, and even forced to take drugs. Today it may be 20%, tomorrow 30% and 40%. Then what? One doesn't need much imagination to see that we are walking clearly in the direction of a drug society. We are educating our children into drug personalities. So, we will have more suicides, more crime, more addiction and more mental problems. Children become teens; teens become adults. Those same children of yesterday are adults tomorrow, believing in drugs and continuing taking drugs. The genetic makeup of the human race will change bit by bit. We will have *generations* of drug-personalities.

A society on drugs is a degenerating and dying society. A drug-personality will flee from reality with drugs, not unlike the person on street drugs. We will have a society with more fear, more toxicity.

But let us ask again: why are we coaxed into all those drugs, even for our children? Yes, the doctors prescribe them and, in the case of mental problems, the psychiatrist goes on prescribing them.

Of course, children are a target market with a price tag of billions of dollars. Here is just one example: the narcotic *Methylphenidate* (the narcotic/ Psychopharmacologic drug contained in products

170 *Haldol* is an antipsychotic drug of high-potency, strong tranquilizer and is used in the treatment of acute psychosis, acute schizophrenia, manic phases, to control aggression, to control agitation, disorganized and psychotic thinking.

171 *Lithium* is an anti-manic agent used to treat manic-depression.

like *Ritalin*, Metadate, or *Concerta*) has increased in Germany by 3591% from the years 1993 to 2005. (Source: Bundesinstitut für Arzneimittel and Medizinprodukte, Bundesopiumstelle, Germany) Systematic marketing (target-market: pediatricians) made this "success" possible. In the USA, the numbers don't look much different.

So you see, there is a brutal, uncompromising market going on – with billions of dollars to be earned! But what is the exact know-how behind this marketing, a know-how that is brilliant and evil at the same time? Good question!

But for now let us read interviews from two experts on children. The topic that is most explosive: ADD!

DR. ARLEN J. LIEBERMAN: "THE PHARMACEUTICAL INDUSTRY ADVERTISES THE MOST HARMFUL DRUGS EVEN TO BABIES."

Before we come to the next chapter and take a look at the brilliant marketing of the pharmaceutical industry, let's hear some words on the topic "Children and drugs" from a top-expert, who truly knows what he is talking about. Dr. Arlen J. Lieberman is today the Executive Director of the clinic "Advanced Medical of Twin Cities" in Golden Valley, Minnesota, where several doctors (including M.D.s) do everything they can to get people well – but without drugs.

Some of Dr. Lieberman's biographical stations included his own Chiropractic Health Center, Golden Valley Sports Clinic, and the Whiplash and Trauma Center of Minnesota. He was the president of Northwestern College of Chiropractic Alumni Association, the Minnesota Chiropractic Orthopedic Society, and the Hennepin District Minnesota Chiropractic Association. In addition, he was elected to membership and granted the title of *Fellow of the Academy of Chiropractic Orthopedists* earning the title of *Diplomate of the American Board of Chiropractic Orthopedists*.

Being a Post Graduate Preceptor, he also uses his facilities as a training facility for students.

"Dr. Lieberman, a few questions first about your background. Approximately how many patients have you treated up to today so far?"

Dr. Arlen J. Lieberman: "Roughly 30,000 patients."

"What is your specific professional know-how?"

Dr. Arlen J. Lieberman: "I am a chiropractic orthopedist and an executive of a multidisciplinary clinic. I have been a pioneer in pulling the two groups, medical doctors and chiropractors, together for the sake of the patients. We concentrate on children particularly. Personally, I treated literally hundreds of children; in my clinic thousands were treated."

"How would you evaluate the pharmaceutical industry today?"

Dr. Arlen J. Lieberman: "Primarily the focus is on big money. If it were to really help people, why would they have all these symptom relievers? They've got all this money – billions and billions of dollars – and they spend it on promotion of those symptom relievers. But symptom relievers don't really help! The best way to look at it would be if you have a pebble in your shoe. You walk around on that pebble, it hurts, and it's very uncomfortable. You could try to shift it around a little, but if you stepped on it, it would still hurt. You could, maybe, take your foot out of that shoe a little bit, right? It feels better. And what happens when you put your foot back in that shoe if that pebble is still there? You still have that symptom; you still have that problem."

"Are there any drugs that really handle things?"

Dr. Arlen J. Lieberman: "I would think so, yes. I don't exactly know what the percentage would be, but my perception is that there are drugs that handle some things. On the other hand, I must say that the symptom relievers, which don't handle things in the end, are probably up in the 90% range of all drugs."

"What are the worst sins of the pharmaceutical industry?"

Dr. Arlen J. Lieberman: "The worst scenarios I've seen is when they promote under the guise of help. Then give flavored anti-depressants to little babies because they are colicky or restless. A child or a baby cannot defend itself or speak out; it cannot evaluate and is at the mercy of the side effects of the drug."

"How do children get into drugs later on? Give us a picture of the whole scenario."

Dr. Arlen J. Lieberman: "Generally speaking, children are a target-market for the pharmaceutical industry. Let us take a look at a child, from the age of eight, nine years old up through the early teens, in school. The child is restless in class, antsy, can't really sit still. And so the first thing that happens typically is the teacher communicates with the school nurse or the psychologist. Then what happens is they make their recommendation and the kid gets tested. Now this kid gets tested and he doesn't rate that high on this test. So immediately they tell the parents they need to see their pediatrician to get medication for their child. But what is really the underlying cause for the child's behavior? Well, the child is perhaps just bored with the subject, has misunderstood words, allergies, too much sugar in his or her diet causing a physiological dysfunction. There are a lot of different things that can happen to a child. In almost every case, you can find one of the above factors causing the child's "behavior problem." It is not a lack of a drug; it's simply a misdiagnosis. But this is the scenario of how the child usually gets onto drugs."

"What then?"

Dr. Arlen J. Lieberman: "If the parents don't comply with the school recommendations, they may threaten the parents to file child neglect or abuse. The facts are that in many schools, the classrooms are too big; they don't have time to individually handle the child, to find out what is really going on with him or her. This I see all the time. Then this child gets a multitude of different kinds of drugs. For adults it would be a stimulant."

"The pharmaceutical industry argues that it is not true that restlessness is caused by sugar. They argue it's just not true that it is the misunderstood words in their school subjects, or that it's food allergies. Don't they plainly say that there are no systematic double blindfold studies proving those other causes?"

Dr. Arlen J. Lieberman: "Let me ask you this: Do you have any children? Or know children? Have you ever seen them after they have had a big candy bar and some pop? You tell me that doesn't have an effect on them? Just visual, following a kid around in a school for instance, let's say they were doing fine in the morning and then they go to lunch. They go to the pop machine and buy a pop and then they have their cake for dessert. Slowly, a little while later, maybe 20 minutes or so into the class period they start going into a hypoglycemic reaction."

"Meaning what?"

Dr. Arlen J. Lieberman: "Low blood sugar. Here is what happens: When you put a lot of sugar into your system. Your body releases insulin. Insulin grabs onto the sugar but then pulls it out of the blood and you end up with a lack of sugar in your system. That is *hypoglycemic.* Then what will happen is your body sees it as a dangerous situation and it kicks in adrenaline. What does adrenaline do? It pops you back up again. So these kids are going through this roller coaster as their bodies are just trying to digest the sugar and food.

"By the way, when you take in too many of the sugars and bad carbohydrates, and you don't break them down immediately, they store as fat and that is why the kids are getting obese today."

"So you say there is a wrong analysis for restlessness. But then drugs are given to the children: Ritalin, Aderol, etc. What are these drugs exactly doing mentally and physically to them?"

Dr. Arlen J. Lieberman: "What happens to the child when you take Ritalin or something like that, is that it actually slows them down a little bit."

"Not rev them up?"

Dr. Arlen J. Lieberman: "No. Normally after puberty it would do that. It is an interesting thing in the body. Just to keep it fairly simple, what will happen is that it will actually slow them down prior to puberty. It will slow them down for as long as the drug stays in the system. The bad thing is that it doesn't always do that. Some kids don't have that reaction, and they will get the stimulant reaction. Most of them though will slow down and they turn into little zombies."

"What happens physiologically to the child?"

Dr. Arlen J. Lieberman: "It inhibits the *serotonin*. It has an effect on the brain itself and how it functions. It will inhibit the firing of the neurons. So it slows them down, where in adults – it acts the same as *cocaine* – it speeds the person up."

"You compare some of those drugs given to our children to cocaine?"

Dr. Arlen J. Lieberman: "Absolutely! *Cocaine* is pharmacologically similar to *Ritalin*. The apparency is that the drug works. In actual fact, testing has shown that kids on these drugs do not do any better, as far as grades, concentration or even in longer term study habits are concerned, than kids that are not on drugs. In fact these kids do a little worse. And another thing, studies show there is a higher incident to becoming addicted to street drugs. *Ritalin* is even being sold as a street drug these days."

"What happens if the child gets off the drug?"

Dr. Arlen J. Lieberman: "When you get the person off of it, you have a side effect of withdrawal which shoots them through the roof again."

"What are the side effects when the kids are on those drugs?"

Dr. Arlen J. Lieberman: "Well these drugs can be very dangerous. Of course, the most significant one is suicide when it comes to *Ritalin* or *Prozac*. Suicidal tendencies, aggression, all these can happen. One of the worse ones for their parents is that they are told they can take their kid off of it during the summer. So they take them off – they go cold turkey on it, but the stuff is still in their system. As you get away from it, the body just starves for the drug and children act crazy. So you have twice the side-effects."

"In your clinic what side effects have you, yourself, seen with children?"

Dr. Arlen J. Lieberman: "Mostly the aggression and uncontrollable behavior. They are running into walls, picking up things, throwing things, and being real rude and mean to their parents and family. A number of them have even gone into other street drugs because of it!"

"You said that even babies sometimes are advised to take these kinds of drugs?"

Dr. Arlen J. Lieberman: "Yes! In major magazines, you open them up and nearly every 3rd advertisement is a drug related ad. "If your child is moody, not sleeping at night, colicky, cries a lot give them a drug. They even advise flavored anti-depressants to babies. So brain washing and obsession really starts early on in life."

"Why is the pharmaceutical industry so irresponsible?"

Dr. Arlen J. Lieberman: "It's just ruthless. There can't be anything but a money-motivated reason to do it. Why would you give your kid something like that? Especially when you know what the side effects are. The pharmaceutical industry knows about the dangerous side effects, yet they continue to push their drugs. That's irresponsible!"

"How old are those babies?"

Dr. Arlen J. Lieberman: "The earliest one I have seen was two years old. But I was told they were giving it to younger children as well."

"Isn't a medicine in general more dangerous to a young body?"

Dr. Arlen J. Lieberman: "Yes, to a really young body it is not funny. One little side note, if you give the same amount of sugar to a little baby as you take in, let's say you both take in a thing of pop, the child is going to react five times more than the adult."

"What are your techniques to get kids off drugs?"

Dr. Arlen J. Lieberman: "We work together with the doctors who are in the know. We work nutritionally with the child. The first thing we do is to communicate with the doctor they are working with right now and say: 'Look, the parents are interested in getting their children off their medication and back into a more natural life.' If you don't get resistance, you ask them to start cutting the dosage down as you start to implement other things such as nutrition."

"What is especially important?"

Dr. Arlen J. Lieberman: "Vitamins and minerals. Calcium and magnesium are the biggies. Calcium is one of the first elements to go out of balance in the body in the presence of an inadequate diet and it is very essential for not only healthy bone and teeth but for stress calming, mental clarity and the nervous system. Magnesium is also beneficial for the nervous system as well as playing a key role in the production of cellular energy. It is involved in almost every biologic process. Then there are minerals such as iron, zinc, potassium, and manganese. Other basic trace minerals are real effective as well."

"What else is part of a healthy nutrition?"

Dr. Arlen J. Lieberman: "A nutrition without additives, without preservatives and without food coloring as much as you can because there can be an allergy to that. No sugar and few simple carbohydrates are important. We work with something we call an elimination diet. The elimination diet consists of taking away those sugars and things for about seven days, which is tough because the kids don't like it when you do that. But you do it. And the first thing is to see if you have a change from just that. You take away a lot of the simple carbs that are not good, pops and the sugars that you know are bad for the child. Then typically you will see a pretty dramatic change, even in their writing. They'll write more clearly. They won't be so jittery. And then what you do, if you want to see whether or not it works or what it is that bothers the child the most, you start adding some of the foods back in and you'll see what actually causes him to react the way he or she has been reacting."

"So you take one bad thing away after the other?"

Dr. Arlen J. Lieberman: "Yeah. You find out what it is exactly. I've had children that were drinking six cans of pop a day and they go through a withdrawal getting off of it first. Then they get better."

"What else do you do?"

Dr. Arlen J. Lieberman: "The other thing we do is we incorporate chiropractic with that. The reason we do this is because the average child by the time they're four years old or so has probably fallen a couple hundred times – fallen out of their chair, etc. It's enough to throw the spine and their nervous system out of whack. So we check to see that they are in alignment and they don't have any dysfunction. And almost every time, we find some things we can work on and that make a significant difference for the child. If you are uncomfortable and you fidget in class, suddenly the teacher thinks you are just trying to be an annoyance. That happens so much. So even the spine can be the reason for unrest."

"What else works?"

Dr. Arlen J. Lieberman: "The osteopathic treatment. It is a cranial sacral technique. It's mostly the cranium, of working with the little bones of the skull as well as the sacrum down at the pelvis area and making sure things are in good alignment so that all the fluids run properly within the brain as well as through the blood and everything else. It's a pretty effective technique."

"You have changed the lives of some children that way? Give us an example."

Dr. Arlen J. Lieberman: "We have had a number of kids where we have gone through these particular procedures. They were able to get off drugs and their grades have gone up."

"You have a lot of success stories with kids?"

Dr. Arlen J. Lieberman: "Yes. When you find the right cause and correct it, the child simply calms down. The parents' stress is reduced significantly, knowing that they are doing the right thing. Doing it naturally, without the use of dangerous mind altering drugs. The parents, being responsible for the child, need to be handled and supported as well. They want to do what is best for their child, but they have been lied to. They have false data sitting there. So the first thing you have to do is strip away the false data and replace it with true data. Just like the doctors – you have to get in communication and talk to the parents. If they are willing to listen, then you can change things."

"What part does the school play?"

Dr. Arlen J. Lieberman: "Sometimes, if they have a bad "reputation" in a particular school, we have them change schools. We do this because some of the teachers have labeled the child as a "problem" child. Frequently, unwilling to give them a second chance because of the amount of disruption they caused in the past. (This is not always the case.)"

"How does that work?"

Dr. Arlen J. Lieberman: "The child gets labeled ADD/ ADHD. It's a disability. The school gets money. So the school is interested in that."

"How much?"

Dr. Arlen J. Lieberman: "I don't know exactly but somewhere over $2000 a kid. It is a really big business. If you get a lot of these kids labeled, you get a lot of funding."

"Who decides that the child has ADD/ADHD?"

Dr. Arlen J. Lieberman: "Dr. Mary Ann Block talks about that in her book *No More ADHD.* Apparently many doctors just take the teacher's word for it and prescribe the drug even without doing a physical exam."

"What other drugs are prescribed for ADD/ADHD besides the ones already mentioned?"

Dr. Arlen J. Lieberman: "Amphetamines such as *Adderall, Dexedrine* and *Cylert* are also used. These are 'speed' type drugs and are controlled substances. And there are antidepressants such as *Tofranil* and *Norpramine*; the latter is stated to cause sudden cardiac death in children."

"Do they help to cure anything?"

Dr. Arlen J. Lieberman: "Drugs rarely cure anything. In fact, they just cover up the symptoms."

"Do drugs worsen the condition?"

Dr. Arlen J. Lieberman: "Definitely. Tests show that after *Ritalin* treatments for eight years, 80% of the children continue to have ADHD symptoms and 60% even got worse. This is documented in Block's book."

"What about some of the side effects of these drugs?"

Dr. Arlen J. Lieberman: "There are definitely bad side effects connected to these which should be weighed out before taking any drugs. For example, *Cylert* can cause liver damage. Long-term use of any of these drugs may have a dangerous effect on the heart, vascular system, kidneys and other organs. Use of amphetamines can cause a wide array of symptoms including euphoria, restlessness, anxiety, tension, anger, fighting, impaired judgment as well as chest pain, seizures, and coma. Even *Prozac, Zoloft* and *Paxil* have long lists of side effects as listed in *No More ADHD.* Parents need to know this before considering putting their child on these drugs."

"How do you educate the parents?"

Dr. Arlen J. Lieberman: "We give the parents facts and true data about drugs. We let them know how ADD/ADHD suddenly came to be. It was voted on. The psychiatrists raised hands at a conference. They asked how many people had experienced this and that. They voted on it and there you have ADD/ADHD. Those drugs were introduced in the early 1980s."

"Again, what is really wrong with the diagnosis of ADD?"

Dr. Arlen J. Lieberman: "Ideally for something to be classified as a disease there should be something physically tangible that you can look at, measure and monitor. Like blood levels of insulin in diabetes. You know the body is not producing enough insulin. It's measurable. Here's a disease you can prove with blood tests, so we have *physical* evidence it exists. Whereas these presumed psychiatric disorders have no physical confirmatory tests. There is no published article that has proven that there is a chemical imbalance in the brain of a child labeled as ADD/ADHD that I have ever seen. The only time that they came up with brain shrinkage was a study done in which they did a test where they measured brain size. They used kids that were classified as ADD/ADHD and used this special type of scan and found that each one of these kids had a shrunken brain. So they were all excited about it – this was at one of their conferences. Someone asked, "how many of these kids were on drugs and for how long *prior* to the test?" Every single one of them was on the drug – *Ritalin* or something similar – for at least a year, again *prior* to doing the test. So it was a bust and it never got published as far as I know."

"So one should make this very clear: there exists no scientific proof, no physical proof or physiologic proof for ADD/ADHD? Its just opinion, opinion?"

Dr. Arlen J. Lieberman: "It's opinion, opinion, opinion. I've never seen any solid data."

"So are psychiatrists fraudulent people?

Dr. Arlen J. Lieberman: "I think there are psychiatrists that truly want to help. The biggest problem is that they have been influenced by their past teachings and influential colleges. These are certain individuals within Psychiatry who are truly suppressive with self-serving, I would consider evil intentions. That's my opinion. And these individuals influence the whole community of psychiatry."

"Why is it that you find those suppressive people in psychiatry?"

Dr. Arlen J. Lieberman: "I think there is a control issue. They want to be in control of and have power to handle everything. They want to be the source."

"How do they convince others of their false information?"

Dr. Arlen J. Lieberman: "They gain the image of authority. They have special tricks in how to do it. One is using big words, using medical terms that nobody understands. And they control the money. They've got the government funding so all of a sudden they've got the power. Then they say, 'If you want to do this, we'll support you if you do what we say.'"

"But most doctors are not so stupid ... they have to be quite smart. Shouldn't a lot of doctors see that?"

Dr. Arlen J. Lieberman: "Yes. But they have been influenced. They have the false data actually put into the curriculum. Through the use of words and big money, even doctors are talked into using dangerous Psychotropic drugs. And there is advertising. There's billions and billions of dollars that the pharmaceutical industry spends on promotion. It gets repeated over and over. 'For your average headaches, depression, anxiety, hyperactivity, this is what you take.' The industry promotes pharmaceuticals so heavily that people start to believe it. It's a sort of brain washing. The good news is not all of us have been fooled."

DR. BENOIT O. CHOINIERE: "A TEAM APPROACH TO YOUR HEALTH."

In United States and even Europe the pharmaceutical companies have targeted children to market their psychotropic, mind-altering medications. Today, a program known as *TeenScreen* has emerged in public schools with unfounded claims of preventing suicide attempts in teenagers. It will label teenagers from a survey of questions designed to "catch" suicidal teens. It has a 90% "false positive" rate and generally results in the teen being referred to a mental health system and started on these mind damaging drugs. In the beginning, parents were not even notified or asked for consent to this survey. Based on a survey taken by children while in school, and often without parental consent, the answers are tabulated and a score determines if the child is mentally ill or not. This is the most recent ploy used by Psychiatry and Drug companies to increase their revenues at the expense of our children.

Dr. Choiniere has been treating patients since 1988. He has cared for many children throughout his practice and witnessed first hand the effects of psychiatric drugs on children.

He is President of Team Physicians of Indiana, PC, and Doctors Plus, PC where doctors of Medicine, Chiropractic and Physical Therapist work together in the same office. A unique approach to today's health care problems.

"A few words about your education?"

Dr. Benoit O. Choiniere: "I graduated cum laude[172] with Research Honor at Palmer College of Chiropractic in Davenport, Iowa in 1988. My Post-graduate studies included Certifications in Rehabilitation, Impairment Evaluation,

172 Cum laude: with honors

Electro-diagnosis[173], and Biomechanical[174] studies of the spine and joints."

"What would you call your biggest success so far?"

Dr. Benoit O. Choiniere: "My biggest success so far, beside being married for 22 years and raising three drug-free and mentally-sane teenagers, is the establishment of health care clinics that encompasses conventional and alternative care together in one setting. When you bring medical doctors, chiropractors, and physical therapists to work together as a team despite difference of opinions and stigma between professions, this would qualify as one of my biggest success.

"How did you get started in your own integrated clinic?"

Dr. Benoit O. Choiniere: "I opened my first chiropractic clinic in 1993. I practiced on my own for two to three years before hiring a physical therapist. We were having great results with our patients, but something was missing. One year later I hired a physician to join our team. For the first time, in 1997, we were able to offer complete medical, chiropractic and physical therapy services to our patients.
"Team Physicians and Doctors Plus have now over 40 employees, including physical therapist, physical therapist assistant, chiropractors, medical assistant, medical doctor. For the last ten years we have been working together as a team to help patients."

---

173 Electro-diagnosis: Electro-diagnostic studies include *EMG* and *NCS*. *EMG* uses inserted needles to trace the electrical activity of muscles and is used to diagnose nerve and muscle disorders. *NCS*, or nerve conduction studies, is a diagnostic tool that measures the rate at which an electrical impulse moves along a nerve. It is used to diagnose disorders of the peripheral nerves and muscle.

174 Biomechanical: the study of the mechanics of a living body, especially of the forces exerted by muscles and gravity on the skeletal structure.

"How many patients have you personally treated and how many including those treated by the other doctors in your clinic?"

Dr. Benoit O. Choiniere: "I have treated over 10,000 patients and altogether, we have treated around 20,000."

"How many kids have you treated so far?"

Dr. Benoit O. Choiniere: "Over the past ten years, I have treated over 1000 kids."

"How does working with medical physicians affect your own practice?"

Dr. Benoit O. Choiniere: "As a chiropractor, we are taught to care for patients without medication or surgical procedures. When I decided to work with medical physicians, I had to keep an open mind. There was an adaptation period for all of us. Even with an open mind attitude, we still had our own skepticism toward each other. At one point, when we all realized that we had the same goal, getting patients better, we were able to actually work together sharing experiences and techniques. I personally learned a lot from the physicians I worked with.

First I wasn't privy to a lot of conditions such as tumors, terminal illness, or diabetes. Because of my association with them, I was really able to spread out my viewpoint on healthcare. It was at this point, the pharmaceutical industry started approaching me with medication."

"What did you know at that time about medication?"

Dr. Benoit O. Choiniere: "Not much. Chiropractors do not get much training in medication, injections or that sort of thing. When our entire department came about, I did my research and asked my physicians questions of what the important points were, what they were trying to achieve, the mechanism of what they were operating on, and what medications were good for the patient and which ones had many contraindications[175] and should be dispensed with."

"How many of your patients were taking drugs?"

Dr. Benoit O. Choiniere: "I would say about 80% are on drugs."

"What are the most common drugs you find these folks take?"

Dr. Benoit O. Choiniere: "I find that 30 – 40% are on antidepressants, 30% are on pain medications and muscle-relaxants, while 20% are on more of an insulin type medication that is necessary to sustain life – like diabetes, Parkinson disease[176], and some dopamine[177] patients. The majority are over-medicated by far."

"What does over-medicated mean?"

Dr. Benoit O. Choiniere: "Basically, they are taking medication that they don't need because the physicians just didn't know what else to do but to prescribe it."

---

175 Contraindications: those things that make the taking of the drug inadvisable: for example an allergic reaction.

176 Parkinson disease: a disorder of the nervous system that affects muscle control.

177 Dopamine: a substance formed normally in the brain that is essential to the normal function of the central nervous system. A reduction of this substance causes certain disease conditions.

"Is it the elderly or the young who are over-medicated?"

Dr. Benoit O. Choiniere: "At first it used to be more the elderly patients, but we are now getting young patients who are being over-medicated."

"How many people are over-medicated?"

Dr. Benoit O. Choiniere: "There are at least 70%."

"In your practice and in looking at your patients, what are the side effects you see from these medications?"

Dr. Benoit O. Choiniere: "With pain medications and muscle relaxants you see patients that are not as energetic as they would normally be. A patient who is on psychotropic drugs will get an interesting glare in their eye as if there is nobody home and they will have some tremors or some jerky motion or hyperactivity of the fingers. They can't stop moving. Get rid of these drugs and he wouldn't shake anymore – not have that nervousness. The drugs were supposed to calm the person but obviously are not doing what they were supposed to do. Or the doctors are prescribing it for the totally wrong condition. I've seen patients put on psychotropic drugs to quit smoking or lose weight. These drugs were not made for that."

"What are the worse side effects you have ever seen?"

Dr. Benoit O. Choiniere: "I have seen a tremendous negative effect of drugs on kids. Even at the age of 11 or 12 years old, they are being put on psychotropic drugs. This is the worse thing you can do to a kid: to create an addiction on a kid. At first the kid will be taking a normally prescribed drug and then if you stop giving it to him, the percentage would be very high that eventually they would turn to illegal drugs. They are still looking for that buzz effect it creates. I've asked some friends who are cops what effects drugs, especially antidepressants, have on kids. They already know what it is. They cannot predict the kid's behavior and have to be extra careful. One day the kid can seem lethargic and the next second he can go berserk – totally crazy, he said. And the cops have to put them down and control them because they have no control, no reality on what is going on, and treat them just like they do a drug addict that's doing crazy stuff."

What about the kids who are not on drugs? What's the difference in how they act?"

Dr. Benoit O. Choiniere: "They are more logical and know that this is the police. The reality factor is there and the police have an easier time to approach these kids as compared to the kids that are on these drugs. Drugs make the criminal more criminal and they lack the reality that what they are doing is wrong. That's the dangers that the cops have seen and were telling me."

"What is your personal experience with the kids on drugs?"

Dr. Benoit O. Choiniere: "When I talk to heavily medicated kids in my office, they are simply not there. I ask them questions, but I might as well ask the moon. They seem subdued, they're calm, not hyperactive which is true, but the side effects are creating a kid that is not as responsive. He doesn't know right from wrong and the information he gives you can't be taken as valid. They are harder to treat."

"What difficulty do you run into?"

Dr. Benoit O. Choiniere: "You don't know what the reality is with these kids. They may tell you they have a back problem, but you really can't take their word for it. Their concept of reality is not quite there."

"Why are so many kids on drugs these days?"

Dr. Benoit O. Choiniere: "Many kids are on drugs today because the drugs are made more available to them. That's the only reason. Years ago the portal of entry for medication for kids was rare and a very small percentage was put on drugs but only for very weird or strange behavior. Today, you get the kid who's not happy and the physician can prescribe a drug right away."

"What reasons do the physicians have for putting more children on drugs?"

Dr. Benoit O. Choiniere: "Many physicians say they don't know when they started giving this drug to a child nor do they know what the drug does. They say they just give it to them because it's been proven and endorsed and everybody else is doing it. Maybe they know the side effects or they think it will make the child better. Now it's a common thing to do, almost to say it's an approved thing to do."

"Who's the driving force behind this idea?"

Dr. Benoit O. Choiniere: "It's driven by the pharmaceutical representative. It's amazing how they push it onto the doctors. Doctors don't know. They don't have time to research it and instead they count on the pharmaceutical representative, who gets paid a bonus the more he sells, to give them an inside of what the drug is. I've seen many of them come into my office and I had to put a stop to it.

I told them they could bring me their medication for heart conditions, or their blood pressure medication or diabetic medication, but I didn't ever want to see a psychotropic drug, an anti-depression or anxiety drug in my office. I don't want any thing to do with them."

"Is this a money motivated drive then with regards to the pharmaceutical representative?"

Dr. Benoit O. Choiniere: "The approach is totally money driven and there's no balance or check on what the drug does. This is a dangerous situation today and that's why we see a tremendous increase on kids being on medication. Unfortunately there is a great marketing strategy behind it and it's working."

"Are there any beneficial drugs that are alright for children?"

Dr. Benoit O. Choiniere: "First of all, psychotropic drugs should never be given to children and there is a lot of medication that was not approved for children. That's the number one thing. I would say 90% of the medication is not good for children. It would have to be an extreme case to put a child on medications. Teenagers particularly respond badly to these medications. This is the age where the hormones start kicking into high gear and they are growing into adulthood physically. It is not the time to mess up the chemical balance at this very temperamental age. It will screw up their mental alertness. If you mess up the balance of the hormones, plus give other mentally mood effecting drugs, you are going to have a bomb on your hands."

"Do doctors realize more and more the increase of drugs used on kids and do they increasingly take the negative

stance towards drugs or what is the awareness in doctor circles?"

Dr. Benoit O. Choiniere: "In my office, they are definitely more aware because I've made sure they ask more questions about medication. They recognize and agree that kids are over-medicated. The only ones that don't agree with that are the psychiatric doctors. Obviously that is their bread and butter."

"Are the physicians in other practices becoming more aware of this also?"

Dr. Benoit O. Choiniere: "Absolutely. The more they look, the more they say this is ridiculous. I hired a new physician the other day and he commented on how over-medicated people were, and he wasn't even sure the medication worked."

"Why are the politicians not more against it?"

Dr. Benoit O. Choiniere: "Politicians have vested interest in seeing the drugs on the market. The pharmaceutical companies finance the lobbyist and since the politician needs the money to be elected, he would have to drum up quite a bit of courage to stop the vicious cycle. There are some that are not in the arena just for the money, but we need to elect more of them."

"What do you think can be done about this?"

Dr. Benoit O. Choiniere: "Talking about it and agreeing that it's not good for kids is a first step. We tended to believe in the past that everything the doctors said was gold, but these days, patients are questioning the doctors more. When it comes to medicating kids, I think that parents need to ask their doctors a whole lot more questions and see if he knows what he is doing and why."

"What would you say would be a strategy to efficiently put a stop to this?"

Dr. Benoit O. Choiniere: "First of all, lawsuits need to be filed. We are seeing more of this these days. People need to be made more aware of what is actually going on. But a more drastic approach needs to be taken because we are fighting a monster. It's like a big wheel turning and it will take a tremendous force to stop it. The pharmaceutical companies have billions of dollars just for marketing. Our resources are limited and we need to get people aligned together to fight this, otherwise our kids are doomed."

"How can this be done?"

Dr. Benoit O. Choiniere: "The more that people realize the wrong that it is doing and the more it is publicized the better. I think we can get a lot of resources on the Internet and see where it is going. We can email everyone and see what the drugs are already doing and open up the communication flow all over from this country to Europe."

"What will be the future of these drugged-up kids of today who are tomorrow's adults?"

Dr. Benoit O. Choiniere: "Right now they are creating drug addicts. The kids are getting used to that drug feeling."

"How does a society on drugs affect the whole country?"

Dr. Benoit O. Choiniere: "A country high on drugs will lose in the next 20 – 40 years. America will lose its leading position on the planet. Because of the poorer education, kids can't read and write. On top of that, they are put on medications that alter their reality and prevent them from knowing what's right or wrong. They won't be able to manipulate new technologies for the advancement of the planet. There are countries that are not on drugs and it's amazing what technology they are coming up with. Take a look at what Japan and China are doing, and India and Pakistan are not that far behind."

"Why are they doing better on not taking drugs?"

Dr. Benoit O. Choiniere: "The reason they are not so much into drugs is that they can't afford it, so that is a plus point. Their governments are not enticing the pharmaceutical industry to produce more products and won't give them carte blanche to implement the massive drugging of their children."

"Does this mean that other countries would surpass us and become leaders of the world?"

Dr. Benoit O. Choiniere: "Yes. We would be left behind as dying countries. Our own technological growth will be halted because we don't have the resources and by resources, I mean our children."

"What do you do to help a child do better besides getting him off the drugs?"

Dr. Benoit O. Choiniere: "First of all the parents have to be on the watch for any kind of mood swing or more depression because there is a time frame that has to elapse before the drugs cease their effect. The second thing is to counter balance the lack of nutrition in the kid by boosting him not only for nerves but for energy level. Electrolytes[178] have to be put in there as well. Get rid of all the fast food. Fast food and sodas are depraved of any vitamins and it has nothing to sustain your life."

"What else can we do to get the kids going again?"

Dr. Benoit O. Choiniere: "Kids today are overweight because they eat way too many carbohydrates. Get rid of the bad carbohydrates such as sugar and give him good carbohydrates you find in vegetables and protein. Too much sugar in the blood causes an onset of adult diabetes."

"What is the best protein you can get today?"

Dr. Benoit O. Choiniere: "The best protein is a good, lean beef but mix it with chicken and fish so you balance it out. Organic meat is better because it lacks the steroids and hormones that are not good for you."

"What do you do with children once they have good nutrition so they don't go back on drugs or the medication in order to get that buzz?"

Dr. Benoit O. Choiniere: "Education is important in this case. You can't tell the kids what to do, but you can show them by taking them to a prison. Police give tours all the time and will show the child what a drug addict does and why they are in prison. They have to know for themselves. What is this guy's future? Do they want his future? If not they will have to stay away from drugs and addictive medications."

178 Electrolytes: electrically charged particles in the body's cells that are necessary to maintain voltages across their cell membranes and to carry electrical impulses.

"How long does it take before the effects of the medication are really worn off for the child mentally and physically?"

Dr. Benoit O. Choiniere: "All these drugs and medications get stored in the fatty tissues and stay in the body for years. Without a good program of vitamins and sauna they could crave that drug buzz in the next two – three years. This means for the next three years the parent would have to watch who the child hangs out with and that he doesn't go for alcohol and illegal drugs. Doing a program to get rid of the drug residues in the fatty tissues reduces this time to only six months to a year. The really sad thing about taking these drugs even for one week is that damage has been done. Research has shown that because of these drugs they will have a reduced mental ability and they are going to begin losing memory."

"Is there some way of finding out if your child is going for those illegal drugs?"

Dr. Benoit O. Choiniere: "Yes. There are drug testing kits you can buy and test in the privacy of your home which tests for five major illegal drugs."

"What are the five major drugs and how are the tests done?"

Dr. Benoit O. Choiniere: "The five major illegal drugs are *opiates*[179], *marijuana*, *cocaine*, *amphetamines*[180], and

---

179 Opiates: any of several sedative narcotics containing opium or one or more of its natural or synthetic derivatives.

180 Amphetamines: a colorless, volatile liquid used as a central nervous system stimulant in the treatment of certain conditions.

Methamphetamines[181]. The test is quite simple. You take a urine sample from the child and dip this little card in it for one – two minutes. Then you read the results from the card. It's called a *Rapid Drug Test*, is cheap and available from us or even on the Internet."

"Do you have a motto for your clinic?"

Dr. Benoit O. Choiniere: "If it's about health, we can help."

181 Methamphetamines: an addictive stimulant drug that strongly activates certain systems in the brain. It is closely related chemically to amphetamine, but has greater central nervous system effects.

5. THE HORROR OF PSYCHOACTIVE DRUGS

Perhaps the darkest chapter one can imagine, when it comes to pharmaceutical drugs, has to do with psychoactive drugs – drugs, in other words, which have an effect on the mind and the psyche. Here we enter the controversial subject of psychiatry, and to really understand psychoactive drugs, we have to understand psychiatry, because psychiatrists define what is "normal" and "not normal," what has to be treated and what has not to be treated, what is mentally sane and mentally insane.

Be aware of this fact: the second something is defined as "insane" one can develop a cure or a drug against it. All it needs is the *definition* of sanity.

So let us take a look at what psychiatrists defined as "sane" in their history. But fasten your seat belt, because here comes surprise after surprise. By the end of this chapter, you will have a *completely* new viewpoint of psychiatry.

In 1758, the first psychiatric book, *Treatise on Madness*, appeared, but it took quite a while until the first universities took on psychiatry as its own branch of study. In the year 1811, the first professorship of psychiatry was established in Leipzig, Germany. From that moment on, it wasn't clear at all what was "normal" and "not normal"; what was to be treated and not treated. Here are just a few examples, which show the dilemma of psychiatry. In 1850, the psychiatrist C. Th. Groddeck wrote about "The democratic diseases, a new form of insanity." In 1854, his colleague, the psychiatrist P. J. Möbius taught about "the psychological insanity of women.[182]

In other words, when a person liked democracy he/she was insane. He/she got labeled as a *crazy* person and had to receive treatment. Another form of "disease" was the mere fact that one was a woman. The fact that one was female, alone, meant insanity.

Unbelievable, but true.

---

182 Dr. Thomas Röder, Volker Kubillus, *Die Männer hinter Hitler, (Men behind Hitler)*, (Pi-Verlag: Malters, Switzerland: 1994), p. 45

From the first moment on, psychiatry also engaged in labeling persons "insane" when they behaved politically incorrect. The famous psychiatrist Krafft-Ebing wrote, for example: "In history, and in present time as well, one encounters a lot of personalities who are not satisfied with the social institutions, who believe the world has to be bettered or that something new has to be established instead of the old...." They appear in the role of the democrats, lead revolutions, create new political parties, sects and cause unhappiness for themselves and other.... [183]

This writing appeared in 1892.

Another German psychiatrist tried to label "insane" the mere fact that one was a Frenchman. He tried to prove that all living Frenchmen are in delirium. Another psychiatrist called the whole of France crazy, "maniac"; another one called Frenchmen psychopathic, giving their "diseases" the name "psychopathica Gallica" (the Munich psychiatrist, L. Löwenfeld, 1914). In other words, a whole nation was designated clinically crazy! Today, one would think that is a bad joke, but in fact it isn't. Later, when we come close to World War I, German psychiatrists called their own German soldiers "crazy," "insane" when they didn't like war. Anyone who promoted peace was not clear in his head, promoted the psychiatrist. Many German soldiers suffered at that time from "neuroses of war" because they had experienced the shock of bombing, lost arms and legs, etc. New words were created by psychiatrists: "Kriegszitterer" (literally translated: somebody who is *trembling* because of the *war*). They also called it *grenade-shock* or *war-hysteria*, *shell shock*, *concussion neuroses*, *exhaustion neuroses*, *gas neurosis*, *nerve-shock*, etc. So someone in shock due to war cruelties was deemed insane! The idea behind it was that German soldiers, in shock, had the possibility to go back to their homeland, something psychiatrists wanted to avoid by all means! So someone who suddenly hated war was sick. Mentally sick. Very practical! Someone who didn't like the "beauty of war" was treated for insanity. Unbelievable? No, just facts, facts, facts!

183 R. von Krafft-Ebing, *Gerichtliche Psychopathologie*, (Stuttgart: 1982), p. 3

Anybody can research this in psychiatric literature written around the time of World War I (1914-1918). An abundance of evidence exists; the facts are unquestionable. So those weak German soldiers had to be treated. But how? With electricity. They were shocked! Alternating current was run through them while at the same time hypnotic military commands were given. Some died, some committed suicide. Even Sigmund Freud was opposed to that kind of "treatment" after the war.

But we haven't even begun to tell the story of psychiatry. Psychiatrists later declared even more people "sick" or "mentally insane" using, of course, a lot of complicated Latin or Greek nomenclature. The purpose was to "help" the insurance companies save money.[184]

"Simulation" in Germany, and "malingerer" or "lead swinger" in English were the new names of somebody who "didn't want to work" or tried to get money from insurance companies. Very convenient! To destroy another's opinion, you simply call somebody "insane."

We haven't even mentioned the real scandal yet. In the Third Reich,[185] there was only one "sane" race: the Aryan, the white race. Psychiatrists differentiated between lower classes of people (not white, not of Germanic origin) and higher classes (The Aryan). All other people had to be killed: sick people, disabled people, even very old people, TB-patients, alcoholics, bums and of course Jews. Psychiatrists worked hand in glove with Hitler's killers. They defined *sanity*! In fact, many of the concentration camps' leaders were psychiatrists. All the names of those psychiatrists are known today and put together in an unbelievably careful and comprehensive research.[186] We don't have to repeat the cruelties of these barbaric historic events. Six millions Jews alone were killed, with the help of psychiatry.

---

184 Röder, Kuillus, *Die Männer hinter Hitler (Men Behind Hitler),* (Malters, Switzerland: Pi-Verlag: 1994), p. 52

185 Third Reich is Hitler's Regime, 1939 – 1945.

186 Röder, Kubillus, *The Men Behind Hitler,* Malters, 1994

It should be clear today that there was only one insane specie here – the psychiatrist himself. After World War II, the Nazis were chased around the world, some were captured, and some escaped. Those who escaped were psychiatrists. Of course, some definitions of sanity and insanity could no longer be used by "modern" psychiatry. But it didn't take too long before some psychiatrists were busy giving *new* definitions to *sanity* and *insanity*. We already heard about the damage they are doing to our children and also to the elderly. One should be very aware of the fact that those psychiatrists use the *same* methods as of yesterday: they just define insanity. With words. With great sounding words. With scientific words. With Latin and Greek words. With complicated bombastic words! Isn't it great labeling a child with *hyperactivity* or any other *mental disorder*? Up to today, psychiatry has a diagnostic problem. The American Psychiatry Association introduced a *Diagnostic and Statistical Manual of Mental Disorders* 1952, revised in 1987 (called DSM-III-R), in which symptoms and signs, personality disorders and mental disorders are described, physical conditions, *psycho social stressors*, etc, are (in the best case) put together, but the labeling of a condition is often questionable. Today, we have less electroshock (at least it is banned in some countries by law), but we have an overload of drugs. We have an unbelievable amount of drugs with partially horrible side effects.

Probably, because of the intense critics on psychiatry and a past full of crimes, this profession tends today to use *drugs* as a therapy (instead of barbaric "treatments," like the cutting of part of the brain, etc). *Anti-psychotic*, *antidepressant*, *anti-anxiety* and *anti-maniac* drugs are very popular in psychiatry circles, despite the recorded shocking side effects. And despite the diagnostic dilemma again, psychiatrists confess in their own textbooks:

"Access to the brain and techniques for measuring and evaluating its functions, particularly mental activities, are still limited because our understanding of the etiology [finding the cause of a disease] and pathogenesis [the development of a disease] of mental disorders is scant.... As a result, terminology and definitions of terms have varied widely among different psychiatrists and in different places."[187]

Nice, how innocent and naive that sounds! Critics of psychiatry, accusing psychiatry of the destruction of human life, simply state that psychiatry is NOT a science, and that the abuse of drugs, up to today, is stellar.

THE SUCCESS STORY OF PROZAC

Depression, that black curtain of despair that comes down over the lives of many, visits over 18 million folks today.[188] Who can bear that feeling of utter hopelessness? Who can stand that feeling of no energy and lack of concentration? It is no wonder that Prozac made such a hit with the medical and psychiatric fields in the late 20th century. It was a miracle – a dream come true. A dream that would soon become a nightmare! How would it become a nightmare? We'll explore that a bit later. First, let's look at the dream come true.

Depression was believed to be caused by a chemical imbalance in the brain and nervous system. These chemicals are called neurotransmitters and are the chemicals that transmit the nerve impulse along the nervous system and in the brain. Serotonin is one of these chemicals, and it is thought that by increasing the activity of serotonin, the chemical imbalance would be handled and depression thwarted. Or so believed the pharmaceutical companies.

Lily came out with the drug in 1988. Its purpose was to increase the activity of serotonin. The leader of the research team, Ray Fuller, was awarded the Pharmaceutical Discoverer's Award from Narsad[189] for the discovery of fluoxetine (Prozac). Bryan Molloy

187 *The Merck Manual*, Merck Research Laboratories: Rahway, N.J: 1992

188 http://www.prozac.com/disease_information/disease_information.jsp?reqNavId=1

189 NARSAD (National Alliance for Research on Schizophrenia and Depression) is a private, not-for-profit public charity organized for the purpose of raising funds for scientific research into the causes, cures, treatments and prevention of severe psychiatric brain disorders, such as schizophrenia and depression.

and David Wong, other members of the Eli Lilly Company research team, also received the awards. It took two years before Prozac became widely prescribed, but by 1995 the annual sales were up to $2.07 billion. That was nearly one third of Lilly's total annual sales! But that wasn't even the peak of its sales. In 2000, it peaked at $3 billion. It had become the popular wonder drug prevalent in the 21st century.[190]

And it was no wonder! Prozac promised happiness in a bottle. And, as it brought the end of depression to many, it lined the pockets of the pharmaceutical companies to the tune of millions of dollars. But we have not yet said a thing here about the side effects that it also brought to the patients, courtesy of Prozac and Lilly. We will take a look at the burst of this dream bubble later in this chapter. Let's cover some other important subjects first such as psychiatry as it is today and the marketing of drugs such as Prozac.

PSYCHIATRY TODAY

Now one could argue that psychiatry today is not the same as psychiatry yesterday, and that all those horror-stories we have heard are only in the past.

Not so!

There is an alarming amount of deaths or even patients suffering from nasty side effects from taking psychotropic medications. More alarming is the fact that psychiatrists, themselves, may not be sufficiently aware of the harm done by the drugs due to the fact there is a lack of reports of these medication errors. Evidence of this is the lack of reports in the psychiatric literature in regards to medication errors and the harm done. Only one issue,[191] written in 1984, reported that 75% of the randomly selected patients experienced adverse drug reactions. What a shockingly high percentage! And only in one report?

190 http://pubs.acs.org/subscribe/journals/mdd/v07/i03/pdf/304rules.pdf

191 Schmid LG, et al: Adverse drug reactions: An epidemiological study at psychiatric hospitals, *Acta Psychiatr Scand* 70: pp.77 – 89, 1984

A more recent study, written in 2002 by Grasso BC et al, shows that there were 2,194 errors per 1,448 hospitalized days. These statistics were a result of reviewing patient charts and hospitalized days. However, the usual method of study for errors had entailed only self-reporting of errors resulting in the report that there were only nine errors per 1,448 patient days. What a variance! This means that self-reporting misses 244 – 1,000 errors for each error detected by other means.[192] One could conclude then that self-reporting errors is not an accurate method.

An article, written in August 2003,[193] referred to a study by Leape et al by saying "lack of correct patient-specific and lack of correct medication-specific information were the two leading causes of prescribing errors."[194] And lack there is! Sounds a lot like Russian roulette with drugs. There is absence of data on medication errors and yet the psychiatrist continues to prescribe.

The sorts of errors that can happen are numerous. A wrong drug may be prescribed. It may interact with other drugs the patient is already taking and create a bad reaction. Or it could be a wrong dosage. With the elderly patient this is particularly dangerous since they are already on different medications for various ailments and their age alone makes it more difficult to differentiate adverse drug reactions from changes in the patient's signs and symptoms.

We could go on and on, but let us state that not only diagnosis in psychiatry is questionable but therapy as well. In fact, one could write entire books on the side effects of psychiatric drugs, and we, the authors, predict that there will come the day when those books will be written.

---

192 Grasso, Rothschild, Genest, and Bates, *What Do We Know About Medication Errors in Inpatient Psychiatry,* Joint Commission Journal on Quality and Safety, 2003, p. 397

193 Idem.

194 Leape LL, et al: *The nature of adverse events in hospitalized patients: Results of the Harvard Medical Practice Study II*, N Engl. J Med 324: pp. 377 – 384, 1991

SUICIDE

The most horrible side effect is of course suicide. Even among children! The Associated Press has stated, "2% to 3% of children taking the antidepressants *Wellbutrin, Paxil, Lexapro, Effexor, Zoloft* and *Fluoxetine* have increased thoughts of suicide." This was based on a study done of data from 24 trials involving more than 4,400 patients taking antidepressants.[195] Suicidal thoughts were most prevalent during the first few months of starting the prescription. The warning on the drug even suggests that the child be watched closely during that time period for any bad signs. And in addition, that the doctor see the child weekly during the first four weeks. Doesn't that speak loudly of the dangers of the drug? Isn't that enough of a warning that something is wrong with this picture?

The black box on the side of the drug states, "There are clinical trial and post-marketing reports with SSRIs[196] and other newer anti-depressants, in both pediatrics and adults, of severe agitation-type adverse events coupled with self-harm or harm to others. The agitation-type events include: akathisia,[197] agitation, disinhibition,[198] emotional lability,[199] hostility, aggression, and depersonalization.[200] In some cases, the events occurred within several weeks of starting treatment."

195 http://www.msnbc.msn.com/id/6254504

196 *S(elective) s(erotonin) r(euptake) i(nhibitor):* A class of drugs, such as fluoxetine or sertraline, that inhibit the uptake of serotonin by neurons of the central nervous system and are primarily used in the treatment of depression and obsessive compulsive disorder.

197 Akathisia manifests as pacing and a total inability to sit still. If forced to sit still, the person experiences extreme anxiety and agitation. In bad cases, the anxiety and agitation may get worse even while the person is moving. Akathisia is dangerous in that it couples an extremely unpleasant experience with an intense urge to act, possibly leading to suicide attempts.

198 Disinhibition: loss of inhibition, as through the influence of external stimuli such as drugs or alcohol, or as a result of brain damage

199 Lability: open to change; adaptable: *an emotionally labile person*

200 Depersonalization: in Psychology, a state in which the normal sense of personal identity and reality is lost

It goes on to say, "Rigorous clinical monitoring for suicidal ideation or other indicators of potential for suicidal behavior is advised in patients of all ages. This includes monitoring for agitation-type emotional and behavioral changes." If you had a bottle of pills with a label on it saying "Poison," would you take some?

THE SECRET OF PSYCHIATRY

Of course, if one looks at all those side effects of psychotropic drugs, the question arises: what about the "authorities," the psychiatrists, who prescribed those dangerous medications?

Well, let us take a closer look and differentiate first between all those pills, between *Minor Tranquillizers*, the *Antidepressants,* and then the *Neuroleptics* (which should be called antipsychotic drugs). And then let us talk about the secret of psychiatry.

MINOR TRANQUILLIZERS

In relation to marketing techniques, the minor tranquillizers aim at people who have one kind of a fear or another. So fear is the trick! The full truth is, that there is none of us without covert or overt fears, meaning that there is a gigantic market here. In fact, with fear as a factor, you can sell anything! There is a conservative estimation that about $800 million are earned by the minor tranquillizers alone.

So here we talk about *Valium, Librium, Xanax*, and also about *Tranxene, Centrax, Konopin* and all those other fancy words that stand for minor tranquillizers.

By the way, has anyone ever asked the question why those fancy names exists? Well, usually they are not understood. They covertly suggest to you that you don't know something; that the chemical formulas of these drugs are so complicated that you cannot understand anyways. In addition, the connection to Greek or Latin roots covertly suggests that there is old God know-how, traditional know-how, and lots of other know-how. And the third trick is that the basic meanings of those words often have a great PR meaning without people realizing it. Valium for example has as its root the Latin word *valere* meaning *being strong*, being *healthy*.

So there are at least three tricks involved with those fancy words. But let's forget the sales tricks and look at the results. What are the effects? Well they tranquillize, of course. But there is also quite a potential for abuse and addiction. Together with alcohol some of those "minor tranquilizers" are lethal. The interchanges with other drugs are not even fully investigated. In any case, when you take minor tranquilizers, the mental alertness is impaired and the physical coordination decreases. The real interesting point is that even those minor tranquilizers can produce "acute agitation, confusion, disorientation, anxiety, and aggression."[201]

Even more problems are possible. Memory dysfunction and brain shrinkage can occur. A psychiatrist, experienced with the use of these drugs, states that minor tranquilizers provide short-lived effects, with little or no evidence of sustained relief. "The hazards are considerable, including addiction, withdrawal reaction, rebound anxiety, mental dysfunction, and lethality." (Breggin, pg. 265) To make a long story short, even the so-called minor tranquillizers quit working in the long run and are dangerous. But it gets even better.

ANTIDEPRESSANTS

Depression has become a household word. It is a relatively new term, by the way, systematically pushed today to get people onto medication. Antidepressants are a multi-billion dollar business as well; despite a plethora of lawsuits that exist against *Prozac*, for example. But who cares? If you earn $10 billion and spend $1 for defense it is still big business, isn't it? Psychiatrist Breggin describes those side effects: "blurred vision, dry mouth, and suppressed function of gut, bladder and sexual organs as well as low blood pressure, weight gain, sleep disturbance, seizures, and impaired cardiac function" (Breggin, pg. 154). Sometimes

201 Peter R. Breggin, *Toxic Psychiatry*, (New York: St. Martins Press, 1991), p. 247

even massive anxiety attacks are possible, and together with other medication, can cause death and suicide attempts. Ha! Ha! Let's stop for a moment. Antidepressants that allegedly help to stop suicide are even responsible for it. What a fake world!

The pill that is said to help a condition can cause the condition? *Prozac*, the allegedly miracle drug, which is currently quite in vogue, has been especially under attack. Some PR specialists spoke enthusiastically about a new generation of drugs. We are not prophets saying that this statement will be repeated over and over again in the future by the pharmaceutical industry when new drugs are promoted. When the true side effects of Prozac were established, one would think one was watching a horror movie. Headaches, nausea, dizziness, impotence, seizures, anxiety, confusion, these were just some side effects. And now comes the real kicker. Murder! And lots of newspapers have stated that!

So one can say without exaggeration that some antidepressants create criminals.

And, boy, it gets even "better."

NEUROLEPTICS

Neuro means *nerves*, *leptos* in Greek means *fine*, *thin*, *delicate*.

The fact is this is the real strong stuff, not mild medication. Synonyms for neuroleptics are antipsychotics and major tranquillizers. In other words, the severely mentally ill person and persons in institutions are treated with those neuroleptics. Approximately 10 million people in the USA are treated with these heavy medications each year.

Psychiatrist Breggin reveals that the side effects of those neuroleptics probably have no antipsychotic effect; they don't heal in other words! But they can cause feelings of helplessness, the deterioration of the mind, neurological damage, dementia, trembling, and twitching, and can impair organs.

Breggin: "Almost any organ can be adversely affected by neuroleptics: eyes, nose, and throat; internal organs, such as the liver, stomach, intestines, cardiovascular system and sexual organs; the skin; and of course, the brain. Be aware of the fact that a small percentage of patients suffer disastrous consequences such as neuroleptics malignant syndrome, sudden unexplained death, cardiovascular crises, seizures, and heat stroke in overheated institutions. These are among the most dangerous medications ever used in medicine!" (pg. 87) Of course, each new generation of neuroleptics are again promoted like a politician before an election. And yet the above are hard hitting facts stated by an insider.

AGAIN: THE SECRET OF PSYCHIATRY

One could summarize that psychiatric pills are extremely dangerous, have many side effects with sometimes horrible consequences, and usually don't work. So what *is* psychiatry?

Fraud! The actual covered-up secret of psychiatry is that it is a fake science! Perhaps it is the biggest fraud that ever happened in the name of "healing."

But why are they so powerful?

Don't forget the roots of psychiatry. In the Third Reich,[202] psychiatrists led concentration camps and killed people. Twin brother of the Nazis. In communistic countries, psychiatrists had helped a suppressive government by using barbaric methods.

In modern times, psychiatrists go to great lengths to be close to political power. So being near to political power is their first technique. It means money. Secondly the masquerade with words, the trick, to use big impressive, "scientific" words, is the oldest trick in the world! But it works! It creates the illusion of knowledge.

Thirdly, the psychiatrists play the authority game. Look at all those impressive doctor and professor titles. By those three *techniques* these guys survive. And fool the whole world.

And oh, here truly is a whole new market!

---

202 Third Reich: during 1933 to 1945, the German state under Adolf Hitler

The United States of America pays $44 billion just for the term "depression" (a relatively new term, invented not too long ago by the way). Forty four billion!

To get people on a prescription, this old trick is used: people have to fill out a questionnaire, allegedly aimed to find out if they feel "depressed." Who doesn't from time to time? New patients are found, and more than one critic has said that this often results in unnecessary treatments with dangerous psycho-pharmaceuticals.[203]

THE MARKET: MENTAL PROBLEMS

Now let's go back to our original cognition: men are markets. Patients are cash cows. New diseases mean billions of dollars.

Let's delve into the thinking process of a marketing director of a pharmaceutical company – one who closely works together with the psychiatrist.

What would be the absolute kicker? What would be the real deal? What would be sheer genius? Right! If we could get the *whole population* on drugs. It would mean billions and one day trillions of dollars. How do you do that?

Well, simply, with "mental screening."

There is a proposal at this moment to impose on the citizens of United States a mandatory screening to ascertain the mental status of every child and adult and to diagnose and prescribe psychiatric drugs. This is the "New Freedom Initiative." And by what criterion will this screening be done? By no less than the worst psychiatric text in the last millennium – the American Psychiatric Association's Diagnostic and Statistical Manual for Mental Disorder.

In this manual are hundreds of disorders, which are actually a list of behavioral symptoms. Imagine finding oneself labeled mentally ill because one could not easily do mathematical problems. Imagine that! This is actually on the list! And there are more of these "mental disorders."

---

203 Psycho-pharmaceuticals: drugs used in the treatment of emotional disorders

What makes this so alarming is that there is no medical or scientific means used to diagnose these "mental illnesses" that is said to be so common. That's right! There are no medical tests done at all – no brain scans, no chemical imbalance tests, and no blood tests.

Marla Filidei, who wrote an article in *The Communication Line* addressing this issue, stated, "With no scientific/medical criteria to substantiate these claims, anyone could be diagnosed as mentally ill based solely on a checklist of behaviors."[204]

The United States president and citizens have been fraudulently misadvised by the vested interests of psychiatrists, psychologists and others into whose coffers will pour billions of dollars. What a marketing scandal! New Freedom Initiative? The only freedom we see here is the freedom of the pharmaceuticals to enslave the rest of the population and become super wealthy in doing so.

PROZAC REVISITED

So what about this *Prozac* dream turned nightmare? Well, it wasn't long before side effects began to show up. It is interesting to note that it takes four weeks or more before there is enough drug in the body to make the person begin to feel better. And once he is on the medication, it is recommended that it be taken for six months or longer so that depression won't return. Mind you, there is no guarantee that he won't again feel depressed once he comes off that drug. But don't worry; the psychiatrist says to just start taking *Prozac* again. In the meantime, he may feel anxious or nervous. Or have trouble sleeping, not to mention lessened sexual drive. Or have suicidal thoughts. But isn't this a better choice than depression?

How about something even worse? Serotonergic[205] enhancing drugs are known to produce the Serotonin Syndrome, which is a

204 Filidei, "New Mental Health Initiative Forwards Psychiatry's Brave New World," *The Communication Line*, Clearwater, Florida: Creative Communications & Designs, Inc, 2004

205 Activated by or capable of liberating serotonin, especially in transmitting nerve impulses

very dangerous and potentially fatal side effect.[206] Basically *Prozac* does not increase the amount of serotonin in the system; it just increases the activity of the serotonin that is present.[207] If *Prozac* is combined with another drug that does raise the serotonin levels, a hyperserotonergic condition is brought on. This condition brings about death via multiple organ failure.

These other drugs can be any one of the following: other antidepressants such as *Paxil* or *Serafem*, weight loss medications such as *Fen-Phen*, or even pain killers such as morphine or codeine or *Dextromethorphan* (commonly used in cough syrups). So what is the chance that the patient might get the right (or should we say wrong in this case) combination of drugs and thereby find his demise?

TABOO: FEAR!

You understand that we, the authors, are not really interested in telling you that *Prozac* is a bad drug, if you understand our cynical and ironic remark correctly. Oh yes, it kills, but the real message is: there are other mental drugs, psychotropic drugs. Psychotropic drugs also have horrible side effects. *Prozac* is just one example.

But how does one solve this problem? Don't those problems exist in fact? Fears, anxieties, depression especially? Yes but obviously the following two statements have never been made public:

(1) Every man has fears, every woman. Fear can be a normal reaction when there IS something to fear. Hardly any person who learns how to speak in front of an audience didn't have fear in the beginning.

Fear is something we consider normal. The biography of the sanest and the greatest of all men demonstrate that fear is part of the being human. Goethe, the greatest German writer, couldn't stand

206 Ann Blake Tracy, *Prozac: Panacea or Pandora?*, (Utah: Cassia Publications, 1994) http://members.aol.com/atracyphd/syndrome.htm

207 http://www.lef.org/fda/fdaban95.html

heights and churchyards. But to label Goethe as sick or mentally sick is a perversity. There are at least 300 different types of fear in existence.

(2) It is a medically proven fact that special heavy metals can cause horrible symptoms of fear, anxiety and depression. Heavy metals? Yes, mercury in your teeth, for example. The fillings can slowly absorb over the years into your body, and cause fear.

The environment today has been poisoned to an unbelievable extent. Mercury, alone, can cause irritability, nervousness, shyness, lack of attention, lack of self-control, depression, and anxiety.

Our environment is overloaded with mercury; more than 40 sources exist, from food (fishes overload with mercury) up to children toys, from which one can ingest mercury. But mercury isn't the only toxin. There is aluminum, arsenic, cadmium, copper, lead, and nickel in our environments today to a degree as never before. They come from the industry, the chemicalization of the environment and, yes, the pharmaceutical industry.

So very often *fear* and *depression* can be reduced to a simple body-source. We will return to this point and to the therapy of it later.

This subject will be dealt with more intensely in a later chapter, so that you, the reader, will lose all fear of fear. Besides there are heavy metal poisoning *incidents* which can be so shocking that people go into a *fear-shock.*

But this fear should not be handled by drugs. There are other natural methods, counseling methods, to free a person from past fears.

So to handle extraordinary amount of fear, one should use cleansing technologies first, which are very advanced and sophisticated today, by the way. And these have no side effects. Then one should ask for counseling technologies. Ask the authors if you wish.

PSYCHIATRIC DRUGS IN THE FUTURE

All those technologies (detoxing technologies, communication technologies) are not of interest to the psychiatrists, despite thousands of success stories exist, including healing success stories. Why? Drugs mean fast, comfortable, and convenient MONEY. Money – that is the name of the game, again and again. The pharmaceutical industry is already earning a hell of a lot of money. Here are just a few facts.

Effexor XR had already netted $775.7 million in the first three months of 2004. Paxil, another popular antidepressant, brought in 246 million pounds to the UK, which is equivalent to approximately $457.6 million in the first three months. *Zoloft* brought in $810 million during that time. And *Wellbutrin* sales for 2004, so far, ring in at $86.4 million. These are only the most popular drugs. There are others to add to the sum that I haven't mentioned. Astounding!

And these all add up to other hideous side effects as well. Paxil has lawsuits against it claiming it to be the cause of suicide and self inflicted harm, not to mention harm to others. In one case, a man killed his wife and children as well as himself after taking *Paxil* for only two days![208]

Zoloft also has been blamed for causing suicidal behavior, and there are over 200 lawsuits filed against Pfizer, Eli Lilly and GlaxoKlineSmith because of this drug.[209] Two hundred! And still the pharmaceutical companies adamantly insisted it was not the fault of the drug.

Effexor XR has other side effects as well as hostility, agitation and restlessness. It can raise blood pressure. And *Wellbutrin* can also raise blood pressure and can bring on seizures, not to mention other disturbing side effects.[210]

And yet the money keeps pouring in from the sales of these drugs.

---

208 http://www.paxil-side-effects-lawsuits.com/pages/sideeffect.html

209 http://www.zoloft-suicide-side-effects.com

210 http://www.wellbutrin-xl.com/benefits/wxl_low_sexual_side_effects.html

Now my dear reader, do you really think that this money isn't loved by somebody?

Of course, we really haven't even touched the subject of psychotropic drugs yet. Because the topic is so scandalous, ten books could be written about it without a problem. Even while writing this book, it was reported that *Ritalin,* if used over a long period of time, can cause negative structural and neurochemical changes in four parts of the brain. (Source: Scientists of New Yorker Weill Cronell Medical College, 2006, 2007) And this same medication is even tested in clinical studies on children who are only two or three years old. How irresponsible can one be?

Or what about *Methadone*, the "miraculous drink," that allegedly helps drug addicts withdraw from street drugs? Well, *Methadone* is currently big business. In some countries, doctors are permitted to sell it to drug addicts, and they also give prescriptions for this extremely dangerous drug. But guess what? Some of those doctors have already been taken to court. One doctor, who specialized in dealing with drug addicts, started a flourishing business by handing out *Methadone* to minors and, even worse, selling it to Russian criminals. Another doctor sold Methadone illegally because he needed cash himself – he was on *cocaine*! (Source: Der Spiegel 41/2006, S. 66)

So what will the future bring?

Well yes, of course, more money to the pockets of the pharmaceutical industry. We will all be screened. And then a drug will be prescribed which we *must* eventually take. Psychiatry and the pharmaceutical industry will make every effort in the political arena, with the help of the media, to sell more drugs.

Will we all be degraded to psychopathic cases? We don't know. But so much we know: NAMES will be invented for every one of those 300 types of fears in existence. Latin names. Complicated names. Impressive names. When Florida in 2004 was plagued by three hurricanes in a row, there was, of course, the immediate discussion of a "new disease." (Because people were fearful.) And then the advertisement will tell you: "*Maybe you qualify for this wonderful new drug. Ask your doctor.*"

But with *doctors*, we are already moving into the next chapter, which will bring even a bigger surprise. First however, let's see what Dr. Whitaker and Dr. Bolick has to say in their interviews.

DR. WHITAKER: "I AIM TO GIVE MY PATIENTS THE BEST POSSIBLE MEDICAL CARE."

Dr. Julian Whitaker, M.D., graduated from Dartmouth College in 1966 and received his medical degree in 1970 from Emory University Medical School. He completed his surgical internship at Grady Memorial Hospital in 1971, and continued at the University of California in San Francisco in orthopedic surgery. In 1991 he opened the Whitaker Wellness Institute, which is now the largest alternative medicine clinic in the USA

In 1974, Dr. Whitaker founded the California Orthomolecular Medical Society, along with four other physicians and the Nobel prize-winning scientist Linus Pauling. Ph.D. A popular speaker and lecturer, Dr. Whitaker is the author of 13 books, including *Reversing Heart Disease* and *Reversing Diabetes*. He is also the author of the popular monthly newsletter ***Health & Healing***, which has reached more than 2,500,000 subscribers since 1991.

Why would a medically trained physician turn to alternative health therapies? With so much money being offered to physicians to prescribe the latest drug via incentives and educational grants, why would any physician turn away and denounce using pharmaceutical modalities as the best solutions for their patient's conditions? The answers may surprise you!

Let us start with a typical question:

"What would you say is your greatest success in your professional life? Is there a specific success you can tell us about?"

Dr. Whitaker: "The answer is simple: Successfully practicing the kind of medicine that I think is best for my patients."

"What made you decide to use complementary and natural methods instead of pharmaceutical remedies for your patients?"

Dr. Whitaker: "I saw early on while I was working at Nathan Pritikin's clinic in 1976 that a natural lifestyle approach to many of the serious diseases was far superior to the conventional drug and surgery approach for treating heart disease and other diseases. So I decided to walk another route."

"What exactly did you see happen in the medical industry back then that you are still concerned about today?"

Dr. Whitaker: "I think the medical industry has become far worse at doing what is profitable for the pharmaceutical industry than it was back in the 70's. Today, we have single drugs garnering almost as much money as the entire industry did back then."

"How about other areas of the medical industry? Have they gotten worse as well?"

Dr. Whitaker: "Yes, of course. The profits and business incentives of not only pharmaceuticals but also of diagnostics have gotten much worse. The increased use of diagnostics such as CT scans and mammograms and surgical procedures—a million or so heart surgeries are performed every year – is far worse than it was back then. I consider physicians to be more dangerous to patients now than they were 30 years ago."

"How about the health care system in the United States? How would you say it ranks?"

Dr. Whitaker: "We actually have one of the worst health care systems in the world. If you compare total life expectancy of a person minus their years of illness, we rank 22nd out of 23 industrialized countries. And to add insult to injury, the average expenditure per person in the United States is more than $6000 a year on health care, which is more than twice as much as in other developed countries. The World Health Organization rated our system's performance at number 37 of all nations when it took expenditures into consideration. When they added efficiency in improving citizens' health, we dropped to number 72."

"What are the dangers you might have experienced for being so outspoken against the billion-dollar industry of Big Pharma?"

Dr. Whitaker: "I've been investigated three times by my state medical board. All three times I innocent, and there was no reason for the investigations. One investigation was actually illegally trumped up by the California Medical Board. They subpoenaed the medical records of a patient, which we refused to give them. The patient had no complaints about me or the care he received, and he denied the board the right to his records. I suggested to the board that we meet before a judge and let them explain why there was a public need for these records. And that case went away. I now have a $2 million extortion attempt by Medicare simply because I use alternative therapies at my clinic.

"Are there risks to other physicians that might prevent them also from speaking up?"

Dr. Whitaker: "Yes, there are risks, and those risks keep physicians from speaking out against Big Pharma even if they're inclined to do so. You wonder why conventional doctors are lockstep in their scorn of natural therapies and dependence on pharmaceuticals. All you have to do is look at what happens to physicians who step outside of the norm."

"How many patients come to you on prescription meds that are actually only remedies for side effects of other medications they are taking?"

Dr. Whitaker: "That's hard to say because we see so much polypharmacy. Patients come in on multiple drugs and, as a result, are doing very badly. Just taking them off their medications and replacing their drugs with vitamins, minerals, and other therapies yields miraculous results. How much of this is due to drug-on-drug interactions and how often additional medications are added to treat drug-induced side effects I can't say. All I know is that the more drugs someone takes, generally the worse off he is."

"How much improvement can be expected when a person is taken off drugs and put on a healthier lifestyle?"

Dr. Whitaker: "As a rule, the more drugs a patient is on to begin with, the greater degree of improvement he will have once we start eliminating some of the drugs."

"Is it more difficult to treat a patient when he has been taking lots of medication?"

Dr. Whitaker: "The diseases we treat in a holistic way – adult-onset diabetes, high cholesterol, heart disease, angina, high blood pressure, arthritis – are a piece of cake; they're easy. But treating people who are on 11, 15, or more drugs is exceedingly difficult. I once saw the chart of a 63-year-old gentleman who was taking 24 powerful prescription drugs. It took my breath away. Now, though that is unusual, 70 year olds on five or six drugs are not. And 70 year olds on more than 10 drugs are not uncommon. So the diseases that are caused by lifestyle factors, poor diet, or suboptimal nutrient intake are easy to treat. Those brought on by polypharmacy are a big challenge."

"From the many patients you see, how often are patients actually taking inappropriate medications for their conditions?"

Dr. Whitaker: "The majority—the overwhelming majority—are taking inappropriate drugs. Let's look at patients with type 2 diabetes, for example, many of whom are taking oral drugs. I consider most oral diabetes drugs inappropriate. The studies back in the 1970s showed that all the oral diabetes medications available at that time increased the risk of heart attack and death from heart disease, compared to placebo. Many of the diabetic drugs we have today are simply first cousins of those prescribed years ago. Avandia® which rakes in 2.1 billion dollars in revenue per year – doesn't do anybody any good and has recently showed to dramatically increase risk of heart attacks."

"Does this worsen their conditions?"

Dr. Whitaker: "Yes. Diabetics are taking drugs that they don't need, which are most likely worsening the problem. Patients with hypertension are taking multiple medications they don't need. The safest and most effective anti-hypertensive drugs are low-dose diuretics. However, patients are prescribed beta-blockers, calcium channel blockers, ACE inhibitors, and a plethora of other drugs in combinations that I believe generally make them worse. Then there are drugs for heart patients. I don't think there's any reason to prescribe statin drugs.[211] At my clinic we stop these drugs on sight – there are far safer ways to lower the cholesterol. According to a

211 Statin drugs: Statin drugs are a class of drugs used to lower cholesterol levels in people who are at risk with cardiovascular disease.

recent article in *Business Week*, statin drugs are virtually useless for preventing cardiovascular disease. The number of patients needed to be treated to reduce one death in three years is over 100. This means that 99 people take a drug for several years and get absolutely no benefit."

"One of our experts feels that only 3% of drugs are effective and 97% are ineffective. What is your opinion on useful drugs vs. non-useful drugs?"

Dr. Whitaker: "It's hard for me to put a number on it, but I would say the percentage of effective drugs is very, very low. And I'm not the only one who feels this way. But I don't know how you could come up with a number such as 3% and prove or disprove it. Bottom line, the number of effective drugs is very low. And unfortunately, some of the drugs that are most effective are not used at all!"

"Is there a time you became suspicious about psychiatric labeling and the use of drugs for the mentally ill?"

Dr. Whitaker: "Yes, back when the first Prozac patient shot up a post office I became suspicious. That was in the early 90s, when I began to seriously consider that psychiatric drugs had the possibility of making a lot of people worse. There's no question about that now."

"What were your observations regarding the psychiatric labeling of mental diseases?"

Dr. Whitaker: "It is obvious to me that psychiatrists simply make up diseases. The DSM, the Diagnostic and Statistical Manual of psychiatric diagnoses, is nothing but a list of clusters of human behaviors that have been classified in such a way as to create disease. So now we have all these diseases that do not have a shred of laboratory or diagnostic verification other than the description of an individual's behavior. They require no measure of chemical imbalances, no pathological signs, no x-ray evidence – nothing is used in psychiatry to validate these diagnoses. It would be like having chest pain or something of that nature and not doing an x-ray, an EKG, or lab work to find out where the pain is coming from. There is no science in psychiatry. Zero. Psychiatry is not just unscientific, it's a fraud."

"What do you say about the testing and radiology studies that psychiatry is reporting these days pointing to DNA markers or brain changes as evidence of mental illness?"

Dr. Whitaker: "What they've done is create a disease such as ADHD and put millions of children on drugs for this so-called disease – and now they're trying to go back and document that the disease is real. Another example is the millions diagnosed with bipolar disorder.[212] Now they want to find some people with bipolar who might have MRI changes. They've been putting the cart way before the horse; in fact, they are putting the cart where there is no horse."

"Today a lot of children are being diagnosed with disorders and treated with psychiatric drugs. What is your opinion on this?"

Dr. Whitaker: "Psychiatrists rely almost completely on subjective symptoms, which are not at all scientific. There are no blood tests, MRIs, or CAT scans done to determine any psychiatric disease. And yet psychiatrists label children all the time with depression, OCD, and ADHD basing their decisions only on symptoms which may very well be just normal reactions to life itself."

212 Bipolar: A Psychiatrist-labeled disease in which a person feels the extremes of high and low emotion. The cause of this is unknown to the Psychiatric field.

"What adverse effect do all these drugs have on children?"

Dr. Whitaker: "These drugs not only stunt growth, depress appetite, cause GI upset, and alter mood, they actually rob children of their personalities and souls. These children will grow up eventually as drug-altered personalities. And there goes our future generation!"

"What would be the effects on society by the drugging of children?"

Dr. Whitaker: "We have already had grizzly murders at the hands of children who were on prescription drugs. We're talking about ordinary children, not criminals, who have committed horrific crimes. Our children will grow up to be adults with fractured lives brought on by the use of mind-altering medications. There'll be a whole generation of adults handicapped in life, many of them acting like zombies or ending up as drug addicts. That will definitely put a burden on society."

"Which therapy used in psychiatry – ECT, lobotomy, psychosurgery, aversion therapy, and drug therapy – do you feel is the most destructive and why?"

Dr. Whitaker: "By far, drug therapy is the worst. These other therapies are damaging and they could not possibly be defended in a rational world. However, compared to drugs, their use is limited. The misuse and overuse of psychiatric drugs affects hundreds of millions. We now have millions of schoolchildren drugged to the gills on psychiatric drugs. We have inexplicable random acts of violence – mothers killing their children, students attacking fellow students. These are not criminal acts per se but random psychotic outbursts, all of which are caused by prescription psychotropic drugs. The student who shot up Virginia Tech reportedly was on Paxil®.

He was under anger management and had been for several years, and you don't get involved in those traditional psych schemes without being drugged."

"How is it that we don't hear much about this in the news?"

Dr. Whitaker: "We don't because the pharmaceutical companies go in and sanitize and threaten and keep information from coming out that would link their products with such insane behavior. So without question, pharmaceutical drugs pose the greatest risk and the most obvious danger. Just look at what they're doing. We have robbed the souls of nearly an entire generation of children. We don't let them mature. If they question authority at all or test their wings, we drug them to control them. They aren't allowed to truly develop. You have to really push the envelope to do lots of lobotomies to create the havoc, danger, and damage that psychotropic drugs have already created."

"What other negative effects can we expect from the widespread use and abuse of prescription drugs?"

Dr. Whitaker: "There is currently a nationwide epidemic of prescription drug abuse in this country. In a report by the National Center on Addiction and Substance Abuse, it was revealed that this type of drug abuse had nearly doubled from 7.8 million to 15.1 million from the years 1992 to 2003. Not only that, but teen abuse of prescription drugs had tripled. In 2003 there were 2.3 million kids between 12 to 17 years old who were abusing at least one prescription drug. This opens the gateway to illegal drug use. Researchers have shown that teens who abuse prescription drugs are twice as likely to use alcohol, five times as likely to use marijuana, 12 times as likely to use heroin, 15 times likelier to use Ecstasy, and 21 times likelier to use cocaine, compared to teens who do not abuse drugs in this way. It is easy to see then that prescription drug abuse leads the way to illegal drug use and addiction."

"Do you have any examples of this happening?"

Dr. Whitaker: "There is a story of a couple in West Virginia who were no longer prescribed OxyContin [213] by their doctor and so they start to take heroin, which costs much less than the black market pharmaceutical would on the street. OxyContin is actually a suitable substitute for heroin."

"With your work on so many patients, are there times when natural and complementary supplements and therapies don't work as well as conventional drugs?

Dr. Whitaker: "One example is Dilantin.[214] This drug is an excellent therapy for anxiety, depression, and a racing mind. Some supplements work well for anxiety and depression, such as GABA,[215] tryptophan,[216] and 5-HTP (5-hydroxy-tryptophan).[217] In many cases, however, Dilantin works better. In certain cases of angina, or chest pain, I don't think

---

213 OxyContin: a prescription narcotic drug used to treat moderate to severe pain. It contains a controlled time-release formula to extend the pain relief over an extended amount of time.

214 Dilantin: a prescription drug commonly used for seizures.

215 GABA: a supplement that induces relaxation, analgesia and sleep. It is a substance that is normally manufactured in the brain.

216 Tryptophan: an essential amino acid that is not synthesized by humans, but is essential as part of our diet and is obtained from dietary proteins such as red meat, eggs, fish, poultry, milk, yogurt, and cottage cheese, as well as chocolate, oats, bananas, spirulina, peanuts, dried dates, mangoes, sesame, chickpeas, sunflower seeds, and pumpkin seeds. It is typically used as an effective sleep aid as well as an antidepressant.

217 5 Hydroxy-Tryptophan: a naturally-occurring amino acid found in certain foods like turkey and cheese used for depression and mood disorders as well as a sleep aid, antidepressant, and appetite suppressant.

anything works better than nitroglycerin. You can use natural therapies to bring down high blood pressure, but you can't always get it down to a safe level. In those cases, low-dose diuretics work well and benefit patients. But if individuals used drugs only after first trying lifestyle changes and safe, natural alternatives, there would be no overblown drug industry. It simply wouldn't exist."

"How about antibiotics?"

Dr. Whitaker: "Antibiotics are useful. But the big drug companies don't put much effort into antibiotics any more because these drugs have such limited usefulness. They want drugs like statins, Ritalin,[218] Zocor,[219] Zoloft[220] or Effexor[221] to fan out to incredibly large segments of the entire population. That's their goal. And that is a major difference from not only 50 years ago, but a major difference in the whole history of medicine."

"Why is that?"

Dr. Whitaker: "Doctors have a history of doing more than good. But back then, there wasn't as much money tied up in medicine. Today we have trillions of dollars at stake, and a lot of money is spent influencing doctors to use specific therapies, including therapies that are obviously harmful. The most dramatic change in the whole history of medicine has been the explosive nature of vested interest. It is so insidious and so much a part of modern medicine that even exposing it does not eradicate it or even slow it down."

218 Ritalin: a prescription stimulant drug commonly used to treat ADHD.

219 Zocor: a cholesterol-lowering medication.

220 Zoloft: a medication used to treat depression, stress, anxiety and many other similar kinds of disorders.

221 Effexor: an antidepressant medication also used for anxiety, panic, etc..

"There has been quite a change in the marketing of medicine – including psychotropic drugs – lately. How did that happen and how does that impact our society today?"

Dr. Whitaker: "About 10 years ago, the FDA decided to permit pharmaceutical firms to advertise on television and radio. When you add this to the ads these companies place in newspapers and magazines, our society is bombarded with sales pitches for drugs. These advertisements always suggest that you "talk to your doctor" about a certain drug to clear ailments such as allergies, pain, high cholesterol, weight gain, etc. But what they really do is bypass the doctor-patient relationship. Today we suffer from an enormous problem of dangerous drug overuse. More than 2.2 million adverse drug reactions are reported each year, and 106,000 annual deaths are attributed to the misuse of prescription drugs. The doctor-patient relationship protects against this type of indiscriminate prescribing, but as this relationship deteriorates, drug misuse will get even worse."

"What are your motivations for being so outspoken against the high use of pharmaceuticals and psychotropic drugs?"

Dr. Whitaker: "My motivation has always been to give the patients who come to my clinic the best possible medical care possible. That's the only motivation that I have. I am not motivated to punish the drug industry. I am not motivated to reward the nutritional supplement industry. I am motivated to give my patients the best possible medical care. If the condition is angina and the best care is not bypass surgery but a nonsurgical approach that includes diet, supplements and a gradually increasing exercise program, that's what I am going to recommend. If the condition is diabetes and the best possible care is not five or six drugs but a lifestyle program, I'm going to take the patient off those drugs and help him make the appropriate changes.

"Do you have any other motto or credo?"

Dr. Whitaker: "That's the only motivation I have ever had in the practice of medicine. I am not philosophically aligned with anything except doing what is best for the patient. That is my motto and credo."

DR. CHANNING BOLICK: "THE ART IS TO FIND NATURAL ALTERNATIVES TO ALL HEALTH DISORDERS"

One of the problems we face today is the fact that the pharmaceutical industry often works via the medical doctors to get patients onto psychiatric drugs. From there, the patient can become addicted for life, not only on one drug but on several.

Dr. Channing Bolick knows what really occurs with patients who are treated by doctors for anxiety and depression. He gives us some interesting insight into the actual situation that occurs in today's society all the way from infancy to the elderly. He has his own Chiropractic Clinic in Maitland, Florida and seeks to find the right natural remedy for each of his patients whether it be nutrition, chiropractic or acupuncture. Along with this, he works with the patient on a treatment that attends the coming off of addictive psych drugs, and the return of health and a healthy life style for the patient.

"What is your educational background?"

Dr. Channing Bolick: "I received my Bachelor's Degree at the University of South Carolina with a double major in biology and chemistry, my Doctor of Chiropractic at Palmer College of Chiropractic in Davenport, Iowa, and then I received a degree in acupuncture from the International Academy of Medical Acupuncture. As well I have a certification in radiology."[222]

"Have you given lectures?"

Dr. Channing Bolick: "I have given hundreds of lectures."

222 Radiology: the study of the use of x-rays as a diagnostic tool

"How do you operate?"

Dr. Channing Bolick: "I own my own clinic, the Bolick Clinic & Maitland Physical Therapy, and I work there together with other doctors, including Medical Doctors."

"How many patients have you treated?"

Dr. Channing Bolick: "I have treated thousands of patients."

"What is your experience in relation to drugs in general?"

Dr. Channing Bolick: "I see that a lot of people are taking unnecessary drugs and many are addicted to drugs who should never have had a drug in the first place. For example, someone gets prescribed a psychiatric drug for a headache – this kind of nonsense. The awful thing about it is the patient doesn't know he's taking a psychiatric drug. The medical doctor tells him it's a headache pill. There is even the case of a person who has a pain in some part of the body ending up taking a cocktail of drugs. Before you know it, they can't figure out why he is so sick; after all, he is taking 13 different kinds of medication, and it isn't really solving the problem."

"Do you know how people become convinced they have to take psychiatric drugs? What is the marketing trick of the industry or the doctor, in general?"

Dr. Channing Bolick: "One of the tricks is to scare people into taking them. For example, someone with a mild case of depression who just does not feel quite right goes to the doctor. So the doctor suggests that they take some *Prozac*. So they start taking *Prozac*. Then the person comes back six weeks later and says they feel wonderful and they want to get off the drug. But the doctor says 'you can't do that because if you stop taking the drug you might have a relapse and the relapse could be far worse than your original depression. So stay on it until it becomes the right time, and then we will put you on a maintenance dose' – whatever nonsense that is. I can't begin to tell you how many people come to me who are on a maintenance dose of *Prozac* or *Zoloft* or some other kind of psychiatric drug and this should be deemed malpractice. No one has a deficiency of *Prozac* in the body. There is no such thing as a maintenance dose of those drugs. The doctors scare the patient into conforming to this maintenance dose thing."

"Do you know of any other marketing tricks of the pharmaceutical industry?"

Dr. Channing Bolick: "I saw one recently in a magazine that had cartoon characters shaped as eggs. There was this female egg talking to her doctor telling him she felt that she needed *Prozac* because her daughter thought her mother wasn't much fun to be with anymore. The doctor agreed that they definitely don't want her little girl to grow up without having fun so he puts the mother on *Prozac*. Well, at the beginning of this cartoon it gives the beginning of the lady's name and the city she lives in, but as you read a bit further, you see this small print at the bottom stating that the cartoon is not actually based on a real situation or a real person. What a clever way to pull on someone's emotional heart strings leading them to believe that they need to take psychiatric drugs for their children's benefit. What it does is play upon people's fears."

"How exactly does the doctor do this?"

Dr. Channing Bolick: "They find out what people are afraid of and then they exploit that fear to sell you this class of drugs. Are they afraid of depression; are they afraid of losing their job because they are depressed; are they afraid of being upset with their staffs or their children? Once the fear buttons are discovered, they exploit it and say they have the chemical solution to their problem. This is how they get their foot in the door."

"How many kinds of fears are there that they can exploit?"

Dr. Channing Bolick: "There are literally an unlimited number of them because it is a personal perspective kind of thing. They just try to find out which one of these are the most common and those are the ones they exploit."

"What are the most common kinds of psychiatric drugs you run into at your job?"

Dr. Channing Bolick: "Antidepressants mostly and the other is anti-anxiety medication."

"What is the favorite target-market of the pharmaceutical industry?"

Dr. Channing Bolick: "They hit very hard on the elderly these days because they may live alone and might not have many friends anymore, or their friends and family have died. They convince them they need to take psychiatric drugs because they are clinically depressed. It's hard for the elderly to die a natural death in this country and not end up on a psychiatric drug before life is over, because somewhere on the line the doctors assume that the person is depressed and he needs this drug. The elderly do not rebel against this."

"Do all patients actually take the medicine prescribed by their doctors?"

Dr. Channing Bolick: "No. A lot of my elderly patients have doctors who think their patients are taking psychiatric drugs when they are not. They take the prescription and wise up to it and throw it away. But the medical doctor harps on this so bad that they actually lie to their medical doctor and tell him that they are taking it when they are not, just so they don't have to hear the rhetoric and suffer all the guilt and pressure all these MDs put on them to take these drugs."

"What about patients taking other medications or drugs unknown to their doctor?"

Dr. Channing Bolick: "People who are doing psychiatric drugs are often doing other forms of self medication as well that their doctor doesn't know about. Maybe even doing alcohol, marijuana, and cocaine. This makes the whole thing more dangerous. It doesn't take long for the person to develop a very nasty drug abuse habit from where they started out with a psychiatric drug."

"What drives the patient to do additional drugs and go to self-prescribed medications?"

Dr. Channing Bolick: "The idea is that if you don't feel as well as you should, there is a chemical solution to this problem. So if the psychiatrist can't find the right chemical for them, they start to create their own little pharmacy at home. The drug industry has never taken responsibility for any of this nor do they acknowledge what goes on."

"Shouldn't the doctors be keeping tabs on what their patients are taking?"

Dr. Channing Bolick: "They don't. It's so reckless of the psychiatrists and medical doctors to not routinely and individually discuss with their patients what they are doing in their life style and what recreational drugs and alcohol they are doing on top of the psychiatric drugs or even take a blood test or urine specimen to see what kind of drugs are in the body; but it is never done. They just keep giving it to them over and over."

"Are the pharmaceutical companies pushing this via the medical doctors for the sake of money?"

Dr. Channing Bolick: "It's definitely the money. There are billions and billions of dollars at stake here. Some of the psychiatric drugs are their biggest moneymakers. They try to figure a way to make it so every man, woman and child, no matter what their age, needs one of these drugs."

"Why is the money at stake here?"

Dr. Channing Bolick: "With other classes of drugs, a person needs them only for a short period of time. For example, if he has a bacterial infection he needs it for a few weeks and then he doesn't need it any more. You also have female related drugs that are targeted for only a certain time in their lives. But with these psychiatric drugs, they try to condition it so that every single person needs it for some purpose at some point in their life; then they try to get them taking the drug and keep them on it for life."

"How do they start out getting them on the drugs?"

Dr. Channing Bolick: "They start out by putting a child on it in their youth for this attention deficit[223] fallacy, for example. And then, as teenagers, they say they are having problems coping, and so they put them on anti-depressants. Then they give the young adult group who has social difficulties and problems in the work place, high anxiety pills."

"What happens when they get to middle age and older?"

Dr. Channing Bolick: "When they get to middle age, they experience depression so they keep them on antidepressants. Then there is menopause and andropause.[224] They call that premenopausal dysphoric disorder PMDD and they re-market *Prozac* under a different name (*Serafem*) to target that group of women as well. They have found a way to position it where it's an unlimited market sector of people that they can pass this garbage out to.

"You get to the elderly and you have people who have lost several of their friends and family members and they get lonely so they give them antidepressants for that. And that is what is so dangerous and alarming about it, and that is why it is so profitable. It isn't a market share that has to be so specialized. You can target everybody on it at one time or another."

"Is it true that one of the reasons for this profitable market is that emotions and bad feelings have never been classified and really scientifically looked at?"

---

223 Attention Deficiency Disorder is a psychiatric invented mental illness to describe a condition in which a person is not able to focus attention, and who is depressed and emotionally unstable as well as disorganized due to some chemical imbalance in the brain. There is no scientific evidence that this condition actually exists.

224 Andropause: the condition in the male whereby there is a lowering of the testosterone in the body as they become elderly, something similar to what the female goes through at menopause.

Dr. Channing Bolick: "That's true. The psychiatric manual, DSM,[225] has never been scientifically researched or studied out. Some of these mental health disorders have been classified in this book by a simple show of hands at the annual psychiatric meetings. No real research or thought behind it at all. Government and private insurances don't believe a whole lot down this line because the diagnosis' that are out of that manual are things the insurance companies don't like to pay for and psychiatric health benefits are very limited due to their ineffectiveness. That's why they have their own separate classification book from other branches of medicine. Every other doctor and physician would get their diagnosis from the ICDE.9[226] book and find diagnosis for real disorders. But these other diseases are so made up and ridiculous that the psychiatrists actually have their own book that they themselves have invented and govern."

"Could one talk about conspiracy here between psychiatrists and the pharmaceutical industry?"

Dr. Channing Bolick: "Sure. One hand feeds the other. If the psychiatrist didn't have drugs to pass out, he is limited to whatever medical procedure he can do such as electric shock therapy, lobotomy and radical brain surgery, and other similar quackeries that torture people's brains – brutalize them. That's all they have in their books, and the public has wizened up and seen the horror of shock therapy and lobotomy these days and aren't supportive of them. Drugs, on the other hand, are something that is socially acceptable. So the psychiatrists are very dependent on the drug industry. If they don't have a new drug to give to the patient, they are out of business."

225 DSM: *Diagnostic and Statistical Manual of Mental Disorders*

226 ICDE-9: *The International Classification of Diseases – ninth revision.* This book is compiled of diseases that medical doctors encounter in their practice.

"What keeps the patient hanging on to taking a drug when it doesn't provide them with a cure for their condition?"

Dr. Channing Bolick: "Let's say a person has attended a psychiatrist for a decade or more and he has been on the current medication for a couple of years. The patient starts to become apathetic or upset about this. They're not getting any better, and in fact they're getting worse. So the only thing the psychiatrist can hope for is that some new drug might be released to solve their problem. One would think that the patient would get tired of it. But so many keep hanging in there in the hope that some other drug that they haven't tried yet will help them."

"So is it a never-ending, money-making story?"

Dr. Channing Bolick: "That's right and that's what keeps people holding on to that line of therapy. If there were only a few drugs available to the psychiatrists and no other drugs being produced in this area it would almost completely ruin psychiatry as a profession. No one would stay in a therapy if the cures they prescribe do not produce results."

"How do the psychiatrists convince the government these drugs are a good thing?"

Dr. Channing Bolick: "The pharmaceutical industry has a lot of money and so they make a lot of campaign donations and people favorable to their causes get re-elected."

"What side effects have you personally have seen with the patients who were or are on psychiatric drugs?"

Dr. Channing Bolick: "The drugs make people worse. I have seen people on anti-anxiety medications who were far worse on them than off of them. These drugs can make these people experience the things they fear."

"How do they do this?"

Dr. Channing Bolick: "There are drug residuals that are stored in the body's fat cells that can be released at a later day into the blood stream whether one is taking the drug or not. This causes a re-experiencing of the effects of this drug – for example anxiety. Just exercising a bit can flush these residuals out into their blood stream. Then they have to take more of that very same drug to try to handle that horrific anxiety and depression that he is now experiencing. So the drug is actually producing the thing the patient is trying to get rid of."

"What happens if these residuals remain in the body or if the person remains on the drugs?"

Dr. Channing Bolick: "Over time these drugs will make the person more and more dependent on them for the treatment. Anyone who hasn't had these residuals cleaned out of their body will re-experience the bad feelings for the rest of their existence. It creates an actual potential for further trouble in this area.

"Just remember, LSD was actually created by the psychiatrist in the late 1950s and 1960s. Congress got all over the psychiatrist and they had to back down on it. Just because the more modern class of drugs don't give as many bad effects as LSD did, it affects the person just as bad and they are every bit as dangerous. They are just a bit milder and coming from a different angle.

"Today most people wouldn't put up with taking LSD for psychiatric disorder. Twenty years from now, we may all look back on *Prozac* with the same hard eye that we look back on LSD now."

"Can you give us more side effects you personally have seen?"

Dr. Channing Bolick: "Sexual dysfunction is another side effect. I have patients tell me they have this from taking psychiatric drugs. Other things are anger management problems. They get angry with family members. The anger was after taking the psychiatric drug – not before. The person was normal, became depressed and got some psych drug. Then all of a sudden they started feeling angry."

"Have you seen other side effects?"

Dr. Channing Bolick: "Another dangerous one is when people take alcohol on top of psychiatric drugs; the anger really manifests in a situation like that. Two of these things are commonly taken together."

"Can you give us an example of this in your own experience with patients?"

Dr. Channing Bolick: "I had a patient one time who was taking *Prozac* for mild depression. One day he went out on a Friday night and had a few beers, went home to his wife, had some minor domestic trouble there and it escalated to the point where he choked her and she called 911 and he was taken to the police station where he was arrested and actually had to go to court – all because of the *Prozac* he was taking. The alcohol had aggravated the situation. Someone on psychiatric drugs who takes alcohol is likely to experience intense misemotion, and things are so unreal to them that they could hurt themselves or another person, and not even realize what they're doing. It happens all too frequently."

"Can psychotropic drugs lower IQ?"

Dr. Channing Bolick: "Yes, it can lower IQ. It changes the way a person thinks and it could change their emotion. Because the cells in the pathway of the brain are permanently altered, it's unlimited to the things that could be damaged on someone."

"What is the first thing you do to help people who come to you who are on psychiatric drugs?"

Dr. Channing Bolick: "When someone has been on alcohol for a long time and quits cold turkey, he gets DTs[227] from detoxing[228]. Same thing happens with someone on psychiatric drugs. They are very deficient on the B vitamins, so they start feeling better once they are taking the B vitamins especially it is very important to take a high dose of B1 – anywhere from 500 to 2000 mgs a day to start with. Another great thing to do is to have them take calcium and magnesium, which are mineral supplements. This calms the nerves of the person down and gets him into a better nutritional state. Repeated alcohol and drug abuse depletes the calcium and magnesium stores in the body. This is why alcoholics fall down and break their hips all the time. Calcium and magnesium do such a good job of handling anxiety and depression that they can often stop taking their psychiatric drugs."

"How does a deficiency of B1 relate to anxiety or depression?"

227 DTs: delirium tremens, which is an acute episode of delirium caused by withdrawal or abstinence from alcohol following habitual excessive drinking

228 Detoxing: the process in which a body gets rid of toxins

Dr. Channing Bolick: "We live in a toxic world and people can have unhealthy life styles, drink too much alcohol, take other classes of drugs and deplete their B vitamins especially B1. As a result, it creates anxiety and depression just because they don't have enough B1 in their system. Any person who experiences anxiety should be put on B1 and calcium and magnesium and see if that doesn't resolve their problem before ever taking psych drugs."

"Do you also give nutritional advice as regards vitamins?"

Dr. Channing Bolick: "Definitely, we suggest programs that are specific to what a person's circumstances are and try to target him in that way. We don't try to put people on a cookie cutter type of program though."

"If you have people with anxiety or psychiatric problems, what other advice do you give them to handle the situation?"

Dr. Channing Bolick: "The bottom line is they need to find a way to get themselves off of that stuff. We encourage them to talk to their doctor and usually we can give them nutritional advice that is helpful to them. The valerian root[229] can be very helpful to help control anxiety. There are lots of natural things that can be done for a person. People don't usually realize how badly these drugs are dragging them down, so once they are off of them they feel better."

"What is your motto for your clinic?"

229 Valerian root: a plant, which is used as a mild sedative to handle stress and anxiety and to aid sleep

Dr. Channing Bolick: "The art is to find natural alternatives to all health disorders. Nutritional therapies, chiropractic treatments – whatever the person might need to actually handle their situation. We provide that."

6. TOP-SECRET: HOSPITALS, DOCTORS AND DRUGS

Did you know that there is an exact PR-insider technology that tells you how to launch drugs into hospitals and into the hand of doctors? This "high art of public relations" contains knowledge of how to influence opinion leaders and key-opinion leaders, how to bribe them, how to get their attention and how to pull them to your side.

We will divulge the exact *methods* of bribery at the end of this chapter, but for now let us first take a look at this hot subject itself: PR! The expression *public relations* sound so innocent, but one should realize that with *PR* whole populations, whole target groups could be manipulated literally into anything. Some of us know the power of PR in the political arena. No day goes by without politicians trying to *convince* us that their politics is right (and the opponent's politics wrong). Not always are the noblest methods used, and in fact there exists a whole arsenal of methods called "black propaganda," a subdivision of PR if you will. But also in business and big business the art of lying, deception and manipulating is known. We know about Bernie Cornfield, one of the mega-stars of public relations. He was the founder of IOS (Investors Overseas Services) who cheated a multitude of people with PR technology. Three hundred thousand IOS-customers lost about one billion Euros in the end. How did he do it? With PR! He even hired the Vice-Chancellor of Germany for PR-purposes and systematically attracted big names, like the son of the former President Franklin D. Roosevelt, James Roosevelt, or Walter M. Shirra, the famous astronaut, the Bank of Rothschild, etc. PR, PR, PR. He put his company into *Switzerland* covertly suggesting with that coup, that the money of the investors was *safe* since Switzerland is considered the safest country in Europe when it comes to money. He continuously talked about making people rich. PR, PR, PR!

We also know how other mega stars of public relations, like the cigarette *Lucky Strike,* were made and built up. *Lucky Strike* opened up the huge market of female smokers with PR alone. How? Well, the PR-guru of that cigarette company claimed "smoking makes women thin." *Lucky Strike* even arranged parades, showing that VIP-women were smoking in public – good looking attractive women who were breaking taboos and thus getting all the attention in the world.

Again and again the company invested an unbelievable amount of money into "emancipation." Emancipation? Well, a woman smoking in public – that meant emancipation. PR, PR, PR. *Lucky Strike* cooperated with fashion designers; PR-specialists created the *Lucky Strike Band* and the *Lucky Strike News*.

Since those old days, public relations are no longer an art but a precise science. PR-professionals know exactly what they are doing and how to achieve an effect. The famous author Le Bon once wrote a book about "The Psychology of the Masses," a bestseller at its time, but today one doesn't speak of *the masses* anymore. "The mass," in a way, does not exist. What exists are exactly-defined *target groups*.

So how does one manipulate the mass? In precisely this way – he manipulate the big target groups. The elderly, children, and sports people – those are big target groups. But how does he manipulate them exactly? Simple. By their opinion leaders. So one has to define a target-group first, and then he has to find the opinion leaders (OL) of that target market. Finally, he influences, or bribes that OL.

Here's another example. The PR-expert wants to influence a town. As the first step, he finds out who the key opinion leader is in that town. Perhaps it's the mayor. But it can also be another mighty or rich guy on whom the mayor is really dependent. The professors Cutclip/Center write: "Each stratum in the community develops its own leaders. The nominal leaders may not be the real leaders. In one town, the mayor is a leader; in another, he is a puppet. Identification of opinion leaders requires probing."[230]

230 Cutclip/Center, *Effective Public Relations*, (London: Prentice Hall, 1964), p. 253

There may be more than one opinion leader in a specific target-market. In a town, that may be the media experts, the influential lawyers, the professors, etc. Once the PR-specialist has identified the true OLs, he has to win them over. In the case of the pharmaceutical industry, this is simple. **Who** are the opinion leaders here? Right! The doctors. So doctors, by all means, have to be won over. But aren't there "WHALES" in this school of fish? That is to say, who are the key-opinion leaders in the group of doctors? Right, the medical professors with high reputation and first-rank researchers are the key OLs. So, imagine, when a new medication comes out, he wins over a *key opinion leader*. What then? Well, he has WON. It is like winning in lotto, $1 million or in case of the pharmaceutical drug cartel, $1 billion. So, all he has to do as a pharmaceutical PR-guy, besides obsessive advertising (which wins the "heart" of the TV, radio and magazine bosses) is EVERYTHING to get these doctors and KOLs in his boat. How does he do this? Well, he bribes them. He bribes them overtly and covertly. He bribes them in a way that can't legally be called bribery. By the way, we aren't saying all pharmaceutical companies bribe these people or that the pharmaceutical industry is only or always bribing. We just say it happens.

At the end of this chapter, we will give some documented techniques of how doctors are bribed, and some general insights on "bribing-technology," if one could call it that. But again, once one has the OLs or even key OLs in his pocket, he is a happy man as a pharmaceutical PR-Guru. He did his job. He is worth millions.

Who, by the way, prescribes most of the pills – the drugs? In the first place, *normal* doctors of course, the MDs. Also the MDs. in hospitals.

So let's take a look at that scenery.

INSIDE HOSPITALS

Perhaps the most surprising facts, when it comes to drugs, deal with hospitals. Hospitals, we think, are safe places where the sick or injured receive medical treatment, good care and help. The word stems from the term *hospice*, a place of shelter for travelers, originally such a shelter kept by monks. Hospitals were once safe places. The term *hospitality* means friendly, kind and generous behavior towards guests. Well, literature proves that many people are *killed* today in hospitals, and we will quote exact numbers in a moment. In addition, ADR (Adverse drug reactions) are the talk of the day in hospitals. Before we come to the specific facts, let us first give some statistics.

Thirty-seven million people are hospitalized every year in the USA In this country, about 6,000 hospitals exist, all together, with roughly one million beds. Total expenses for all USA registered hospitals are $570,534,159,000.[231] Roughly spoken, 570 billion or very roughly, over half a trillion dollars! About 40% of health care expenditures in the USA go towards hospitals; hospitals are the big part when it comes to cost. Five of the top ten conditions for which people are admitted to the Emergency room are heart problems, like heart attack; two of the top ten conditions are infections: pneumonia and blood infection. Depression also belongs in the top ten conditions treated. The average charge for a hospital stay is over $11,000.[232] Usually hospitals are owned by a group of doctors.

So far, nothing is wrong with those statistics. We still tend to believe that hospitals are safe places. But listen to this fact: people *die* today for no other reason than *being* in a hospital. And not in small numbers. The actual numbers differ from source to source: "195,000 USA deaths blamed on hospital errors,"[233] says Reuters. The JAMA publication (Journal of the American Medical Association) talks about 106,000 deaths caused by negative effects of drugs every year.[234] Harvard University again has different numbers and according to the Albuquerque Journal, in relating to

231 http://www.aha.org/aha/content/2006/pdf/fastfacts2006.pdf

232 Agency for Healthcare Research and Quality

233 Source: Reuters, updated: July 28, 2004

234 Source: *http://www.alkalizeforhealth.net/Ldoctordeath.htm*

a federal study, talks about 44,000 to 98,000 people who die each year in hospitals because of errors, 20% of which were due to medication slips-ups."[235] But the number of 195,000 people who die in the USA each year seems to be the most reliable and most quoted number.[236]

Again: 195,000. Dead!

We did not mention the fact that very often people are in hospitals undergoing unnecessary surgery. Surgeons love to operate in the case of back pain, heart or knee problems. And the statistics are rising dramatically. In Germany, 65 thousand patients had surgery in 1998 because of disc-problems. In 2003, 100 thousand. As far as we could research it, there were even more in 2007. And this despite the fact that in 90% of the cases the pain goes away by itself.[237] Let us repeat: 90%!

Financial interests of the surgeons and/or the hospitals are often the key. Critics state that in only one case out of seven enough data is gathered to justify an operation (Spiegel 35/2005, pg. 135).

And here is the kicker. In the spring of 2000, Israeli hospital doctors of Jerusalem went on strike for many weeks. Tens of thousands of operations did not take place. Only emergency clinics, etc. stayed open. The result? A survey was made in the mortuaries where the hospitals were closed. Guess what? People died less. (Jörg Blech, in: Der Spiegel, 35/2005 pg 143) Needless to say that before, during and after the operation, many different drugs are used. What a big business!

There are hardly any systematic studies available; of course, the subject is too embarrassing for the medical authorities. *Death* is the worst-case scenario, but it does happen without any doubt in hospitals today. Even literature in relation to that already exists.

---

235 See http://md-jd.info/iom-011.htm and http://www.nypirg.org/patientsafety/medication.pdf

236 See updated study of Jennifer Warner, "Medical Errors Still Plague USA hospitals," http://women.webmd.com/news/20040727/medical-errors-plague-us-hospitals

237 In Germany alone, 52 thousand "medications" are on the market despite that WHO states that only 306 are really necessary.

Author May Lorrie Davis wrote a book entitled *How to Survive a Stay in the Hospital without Getting Killed.* The title says it all.

But drugs in hospitals also can cause ADR (Adverse Drug Reaction). One should never forget that especially elderly people end up in hospitals. They usually take a large amount of drugs already. Those drugs can interact. When new drugs are added the most horrible side effects are possible. We predict there will be a new *science* one day that will deal just with the interaction of drugs alone. Some interactions can be deadly; some can lead to more or less serious side effects.

In addition to the interaction, it can also be the case that the *wrong* drug is given. And it can be that an *overdose* is prescribed. Also drugs can be given at the *wrong time.*

Experts differentiate between relatively non-dangerous side effects (such as mild drowsiness), the harder side effects (such as chronic cough) and serious side effects (hemorrhage). Death is the ultimate "side effect."

So, it is not only alarming, that a huge number of people are hospitalized today *because* of the side effects of drugs (wrong medicine, wrong doses, etc), but when one is in a hospital, additionally he can be the victim of medical errors.

How many ADRs exist today in the United States hospitals? Well, the American Medical Association, for sure not a drug-enemy, talks about "2.2 million adverse drug reactions among hospitalized patients nationwide."[238] Yes, all sorts of drugs are included, but drugs are drugs.

So we are *not* talking here about faulty diagnosis, the use of outmoded tests, equipment failure, surgery on the wrong limb or organ tissue samples lost or misread, an object left inside a patient during surgery, or mistaken patient identities. "By far the most common problem is when patients receive incorrect dosages or types of medications.... Prescriptions are unreadable or vague, the right medication is given to the wrong patient or different medicines

238 http://www.heall.com/body/healthupdates/drugs/adversedrugs.html

have a bad interaction."[239] Shall I put it clearer? OK. "There is a one in 15 chance that you will have an adverse reaction to a drug in a hospital."[240]

So what is the problem here?

One should remember that even over-the-counter medicines and herbs could interact with drugs, and yes, even Vitamins, minerals, supplements and homeopathic preparations. So it is not only the high doses, the powerful drug or the wrong drug, it is the *interaction* of drugs with drugs and other substances. Authors trying to help patients in hospitals advise them to name a health care surrogate or advisor before entering a hospital. Some time back, *The Washington Post* talked about plastic identity bracelets with bar codes containing information to make sure patients do not get the wrong drug or dosage by mistake. Other authors advise us to look for ourselves, judge for ourselves, but all this advice forgets one point: we take, *by far,* too many drugs in general.

It takes quite a while until a dangerous drug is taken off the market, and how many *new* drugs are invented every year. Because long-term studies are missing in most of the cases, this makes the situation in hospitals even more dangerous.

So what will be the future in our hospitals? Imagine the increasing number of drugs. Imagine that more and more drugs are taken. Imagine that the interaction of drugs have, in many cases, not been tested sufficiently. So what will the future bring? Yes, we will have more side effects. To get the exact numbers of death and ADR will be more and more difficult, because it puts a light on our hospitals, which is not very bright. And medical authorities will not be very eager to put the correct data together. Perhaps we will have in the future two *types* of hospitals (partially this is already the case), hospitals with alternative medicine and lots of care, elite hospitals and the "normal" hospital. Truths about our hospitals

---

239 Tom Clavin, "How you can protect yourself," May 23, 2004, http://www.parade.com/articles/editions/2004/edition_05-23-2004/featured_0

240 Dr. Joseph Mercola, "Serious and Fatal Drug reactions in USA Hospitals," http://articles.mercola.com/sites/articles/archive/2008/01/02/hospital-drug-reactions.aspx

are beginning to spread. We will probably find first-class, natural treatment hospitals and hospitals with drug-treatments.

So let us repeat: first, many people end up in the hospitals *because* of drugs. And then they have to fight drugs again *in* the hospital.

Now let us go back to our original theme: bribery.

BRIBERY

Just imagine, bribery by the pharmaceutical industry has even been documented in literature. One doesn't even have to fear the lawyer stating that (direct or indirect) bribery took place. Bribery is always very covert, very secretive, very hidden, right? Wrong. There are sublime methods of giving first a *little* something which really can't be called bribery, then giving a *little* bit more, then a little bit more and more … you understand? One can lure somebody, step by step, into *liking* a company. Who can be against a bottle of champagne for example? Who can say anything against a Havana? One should know that there is a *high* art of bribery. How is it done? To smartly bribe a person, one finds out what people respond to, what motivates them. Well, people can be, in general, motivated by decorations, honors, prizes, titles, money, precious objects and traveling. A whole *science* of motivation exists here already. To efficiently bribe (read: motivate) a target group one finds out the primary motivation of that target group.

What is the primary motivation of doctors? Guess. Well, objective surveys found that out: *money!* Doctors, in general, are motivated by money; they are (in general) not motivated by the urge to help people. Most doctors are doctors because they can make a good living with their jobs. (Teachers, by the way, are not motivated by money, they usually like to educate and help children. Insurance and sales people are also motivated, usually, by money. Traveling possibilities motivates Stewardess', who like to fly and see the world.

To efficiently motivate doctors a person has to give them *money* or money-like advantages. How does one give them money-like advantages? Well, by giving them a computer-network for example. The following information is taken mostly from the transcript of a Senate hearing before the *Senate Committee on Labor and Human Resources,* chaired by Senator Edward Kennedy. The primary testimony is by Dr. Sidney Wolfe, M. D. director of the *Public Citizens Health Research Group*, non-profit watchdog of the drug industry.

The most outrageous case of bribery that Dr. Wolfe found was executed by a company called Physicians Computer Network (PCN). This company was really a front organization for the 10 largest drug companies.

PCN gave doctors big, elaborate "practice management" software and hardware packages that computerize details on every patient, the diagnosis, and the drugs prescribed, and does billing and other bookkeeping chores.

There were two conditions necessary to receive this equipment: one, allow PCN to hook it to a phone modem so they can access the information anytime (except for name and address of the patient); and two, the doctor must watch 32 ads a month that appear on this computer system and answer one clinically oriented question per ad. Now that's very cheap conditions for a $35,000.00 system. Wouldn't you say? It means about 32 minutes of the doctor's time per month.[241]

Smart? Of course, very smart from the viewpoint of the drug company. The drug company gets marketing information, gets info about the doctors and forces them to look at their medication/drugs advertisement.

Another example: *Roche* paid $1,200.00 cash for prescribing expensive antibiotics – paid to the pharmaceutical industry. Doctors were asked to participate in a "clinical study." Oh, how nice and innocent one can express that. In this "clinical study" a synthetic

241 *Amazing Medicines the Drug Companies Don't Want You to Discover*! (Medical Research Publishers Tempe, Arizona, 1993,) p. 14

variant of penicillin had to be given to patients. The "exchange" was $1,200.00 dollars.

Another example: free flights were offered by drug company *Wyeth-Ayerst*. Fifty prescriptions meant a free ticket to anywhere in the USA.[242]

Another example: gourmet dinners. The value is sometimes as much as $200. During this *gourmet dinner* the doctor listens to lectures, to new information; he gets drugs sold, in other words.

Of course it is not called bribery, oh no!

Another example: doctors get *points* for prescription of special drugs, as in the case of *Connaught Laboratories*. In the end, with enough points, the doctor gets a video camera, a computer, a TV or medical equipment.[243] Nice! Shall we go on?

DER SPIEGEL reported (28/2004) that Pharma-producer Sandoz tried to pay commissions to *health-nets*, which consist of doctors.

The whole game is called "incentives." As stated earlier, how to *motivate* is a whole art today, played by the PR industry. Of course it all gets done so that the image of *bribery* does not exist.

Here is another sophisticated technique. Imagine a TV-boss (somebody who decides what features get shown) being *convinced* by the pharmaceutical company to show a special (good) feature. How is it done? The high art, of course, consists of researching what this TV-director really likes. Even more sophisticated is this: one invites this TV-director to give a speech to the pharmaceutical company. There is nothing wrong with this, is it? Of course not. Anybody can give a speech to a pharmaceutical company. Oh, we just forgot to say that this speech or lecture is honored with $10,000 dollars. So even this is totally legal. *Honi soit qui mal y pense* only a rogue can think there is something wrong. Or? To say it sarcastically, the good old days where one gives a person CASH are partially over. Since politicians have been bribed by Arabian countries and photographed receiving money (a bribe-trap), this

242 Ibid. p. 16

243 Ibid. p. 18

type of bribery is OUT. That is not the high art anymore. There is a finer art of bribery that is not considered illegal or dangerous. The fine art is: MANUS MANUM LAVAT. One hand washes the other hand. It can't even legally be called bribery anymore, you see? It would have to be called "motivation." Isn't that sly!

Only one state in the USA has a law against doctor bribery, and this is Massachusetts.

Criminal investigations have been launched against pharmaceutical bribery, but one can be sure that this is just the tip of the iceberg. Free airline tickets, free diagnostic equipment, even a money loan with low interest to build up the doctor's office in the beginning of his career (often found in Germany) – all these things happened. This and more have been offered by pharmaceutical companies to win over doctors. And the doctor, who is usually "motivated" by money, what will he do? Yes, he will take the advantages and put people on drugs.

If one thinks that he now has a pretty good picture of the pharmaceutical industry, he errs again. There is more in relation to lying, to black propaganda-techniques and hiding the truth. So, let us just take a look at another prominent target group: the athletes, after the following interview.

DR. JOHN T. FEULNER, DPM:[244] "DRUGS AND SURGERY ARE IN MANY CASES UNNECESSARY TO HANDLE PAIN."

Drugs, drugs, drugs! Drugs are also used to an unbelievable degree in surgery today despite the fact that professionals know about the side effects they cause. What many people don't know is the fact that in many cases a surgical operation can, in fact, be avoided.

Let us take a look at just one subject. Podiatric Medicine…

These days it is not uncommon to hear of people undergoing knee and hip replacements so that they can walk again. In 2002 alone, there were 193,000 hip replacements and that statistic has gone up considerably for 2005. This involves surgery and drugs and is not always the best solution to say the least. As well, 10% of these patients return for further surgery on the same knee or hip. And here is the amazing news. There is an alternative that does not involve surgery and does not use drugs and which produces excellent results in reducing pain and enabling the patient to walk again.

But *how* is that done? To find out we interviewed, for this book, a top-expert who is specialized in handling the basic cause of degenerating knees and hips. Dr. John T. Feulner was a member of the National Athletics Trainers' Association from 1988 – 2002, but also, not only operates the *Florida Biomechanics Clinic* with his partner Dr. Robert Levine, but is the owner of *Foot Doc Orthotic Labs* where he makes the orthotic arch supports and braces for an imbalanced skeletal structure. Both the clinic and the lab are synergistic, meaning that together they are more effective than they would be on their own. Dr. Feulner does not recommend surgery but instead achieves amazing successes usually using his own technology for balancing the skeletal system. But how does he achieve that? Let's research a bit further and jump right into the middle of the interview.

---

244 DPM: Doctor of Podiatric Medicine

"What is your educational background?"

Dr. John Feulner: "In the mid 80s I attended four years at the *Kean College* of New Jersey and became a Certified Athletic Trainer. Then I attended four years at the *New York College of Podiatric Medicine* and received my doctorate as a Podiatrist. I also went to *North Western University* in Chicago and completed an advanced orthotics program. After doing a one and a half year residency program in orthotics and another year in Podiatry, I became fully trained in all sorts of brace making as well as in podiatric medicine and surgery. I was not interested in doing surgery, so I took a job working with a company for seven years making orthotic arch supports."

"What would you say was your biggest success?"

Dr. John Feulner: "My biggest success has been to master the technology that I and my partner utilize to fix the body's aches and pains well over 95% of the time. If you can manipulate and affect the skeleton's position, you will affect the muscle balance and if the muscles balance correctly, the joints move easily and smoothly. Subsequently they don't grind and prematurely erode or destroy the ends of the bones."

"Why choose the feet?"

Dr. John Feulner: "A large percentage of the population has something called over-pronation[245] which is a condition where the arch collapses, the heels tilt outward and the shin bone rotates inwardly. In more severe cases, the inside anklebone becomes more pronounced. The more the arches

245 Pronation: the turning or rotating of the foot so that the inner edge of the sole bears the body's weight

are flattened the more those three things happen. Excessive inward shin rotation places torque directly on the knee joint which starts to place undue stress on the ligaments and bones that make up the joint."

"What is the cause for all these problems the bodies are having with knees and hips today?"

Dr. John Feulner: "One hundred years ago, we were not walking on any one particular surface; there were a variety of surfaces. More recently, we have been predominately walking on concrete; a hard but more importantly, a completely flat surface. We get up in the morning and step onto hardwood floors that are laid on top of concrete, walk into the bathroom, which has tiles on top of concrete. Once outside the house we walk on sidewalks that are concrete and into our car. Parking the car in a concrete parking lot, we walk over to a building which has a floor also made of concrete, having usually thin carpet laid over top. Rarely do we step off this walking surface."

"What are the ramifications besides the fact it is hard and unyielding?"

Dr. John Feulner: "On this completely flat surface we only function in one position. If you were alive 200 plus years ago, you would be walking on varied terrains up and down uneven hills, through fields and over rocks so the foot was forced to operate in a functional range of motion and subsequently maintained strength around dozens of different positions. Because of this, the foot maintained a better flexibility and a better range of motion because if you don't use it, you lose it. The point is that form follows function. When you put a normal healthy arm into a cast for eight to ten weeks, you would find that it would have very little strength and very little motion once the cast is removed. So, due to the fact that we walk almost exclusively on a hard flat unyielding surface, our feet and subsequently the body only functions in that one position. So we build strength in a range of motion mainly around that one position. That's why we are so weak muscularly in so many different positions and that's primarily why we have a lack of shock absorption."

"How do you develop shock absorption?"

Dr. John Feulner: "The way to get shock absorption is to keep oneself in the middle of a range of motion. If you are at the beginning of a range of motion and you are held there, there is no motion so there is no shock absorption. If the arch flattens out and stays like that, we function at the end of a range of motion. When you function at the end of a range of motion there is no shock absorption. That's why we have all these orthopedic problems. The literature expounds on well over thirty specific diagnosis, all kinds of knee pathology,[246] ankle problems, fallen arches, plantar fasciitis,[247] bunions,[248] hammer toes,[249] and lower back stuff that all relate to a single etiology, a common factor, and that is over-pronation[250] which is basically the collapsing of the arches."

246 Pathology: the anatomy of functional manifestations of a disease

247 Plantar fasciitis: heel pain caused by various things such as inadequate flexibility in the calf muscles, lack of arch support, being overweight, suddenly increasing activity, and spending too much time on the feet

248 Bunion: a painful, inflamed swelling of the bursa (a sac or sac-like cavity containing lubricating fluid between the joint and tendon) at the first joint of the big toe, characterized by the enlargement of the joint and displacement of the toe

249 Hammertoes: toes, usually the second ones that are permanently flexed downward, resulting in a claw-like shape

250 Over-pronation: the turning or rotating of the foot so that the inner edge of the sole bears the body's weight, flat feet

"Do you teach how to walk correctly?"

Dr. John Feulner: "What we do is something called Gait Analysis.[251] As I watch the way someone walks, I can spot imbalances. When a person's arches are flat, especially when one is more flat than the other, the first concept is that it affects the entire body. This is the first stable datum. It creates rotation in the bones of your body that is more that the normal rotation should be. Therefore, it adversely affects all the joints and muscles in the body. The trick is to be expert in spotting the imbalances. You can tell one arch is lower than the other when people stand; one foot points in one direction and the other points in a totally different direction etc..."

"What other technologies exist that address the body's imbalances?"

Dr. John Feulner: "In my opinion, very few technologies are as effective in addressing this situation because they miss the right reason for the imbalance. Just like drugs, they can mask the symptoms. Many times practitioners treat the symptoms and don't look at the basic cause and what's actually causing the knee pain. They suggest doing surgery on the knee, for example. But it's not the knee that is the problem. It began with the feet."

"Among all the different philosophies of handling the body, what are the correct ones?"

Dr. John Feulner: "There are many different philosophies that claim to treat this imbalance, but the field of biomechanics is muddied with inconsistent results. Because of this, corrective arch supports and other orthotic devices have been given a

251 Gait analysis: the study of how a person walks

bad name due to the amount of overall inconsistency. Our technology is consistent and predictable because we get a very high success rate; as I said earlier, over 95% of the time."

"How about the body building trainers; what is their thought on this?"

Dr. John Feulner: "In general, the trainers feel that they can support and control the foot's arch by strengthening the muscles that control the arch."

"Isn't muscle training important?"

Dr. John Feulner: "Yes, but I don't agree with that fully. It's part of it, but structurally, if the skeleton is not in a sound position a person can strengthen muscles all he wants but the structural misalignment is going to ultimately overpower the muscles every single time. Muscle balance and muscle strengthening is key to proper function, but the bottom line is, the structural components which aligns the skeletal structure has to be addressed first. If he can keep the skeleton in good structural alignment, then, yes, muscle strengthening is very important, but if he cannot maintain that good structural alignment he will never get rid of his joint and muscle pains."

"Should the patient also go to a chiropractor?"

Dr. John Feulner: "Going to a chiropractor can definitely be part of the solution. The point here is that the skeletal alignment must be stably maintained for chiropractic or any treatment or any other treatment modality to be effective. This of course includes surgery when absolutely necessary"

"Why is that?"

Dr. John Feulner: "If there is a basic structural imbalance so that when one foot collapses too much, for example, it will throw the rest of the skeletal system out. This is how it works. A significantly lowered arch will result in excessive inward shinbone rotation. If that occurs to different degrees in each leg because of an asymmetric imbalance, the excessive torque will be more severe on one leg and knee more than the other. This then causes the upper leg and thighbone to rotate inwardly which then rotates and tilts the pelvis, usually unevenly. That's what causes lower back pain and all kinds of problems all the way up the entire skeletal structure. Again, the point here is to address the structural alignment first."

"Do you work along with the chiropractors?"

Dr. John Feulner: "Yes. We work along with chiropractors because if we keep the structural alignment of the skeleton in good position, the muscles can then be effectively strengthened and optimal function can be restored.

"What are the most problems you run into with the people who come to you?"

Dr. John Feulner: "Some people we get are those who suffer from any of the joint arthritis ailments – the painful stuff – the degenerative joint disease also known as osteoarthritis.[252] It's mechanical. It's from uneven joint wear.

"We also get quite a few people who are into physical fitness. Since we are raising people's awareness to the fact that the foot is the gatekeeper for the entire body, we get folks who wish to become more fit or who wish to get to the

---

252 Osteoarthritis: a form of arthritis, usually in older people, in which the cartilage in the joints is worn down

next level of training but because of muscle aches and pains, just cannot. This is because the foot may be preventing their fitness goals. People with chronic sports injuries and people with chronic fatigue have to alter their life styles. They can't do the things they want to do. They go to the gym and hurt themselves because of the imbalance. Trainers are plagued with that. They get people who want to improve their bodies but they get hurt and can't. Many times they are advised anti-inflammatory or pain meds and they stop training altogether. With athletes, this is an emotional thing because when athletes can't do what they want to do, it is devastating. It's a life purpose. Some get steered by psychiatrists to take psychotropic drugs because they are depressed. People take advantage of this at every turn. It is disgusting."

"Do regular folks come to see you also?"

Dr. John Feulner: "Yes. People who are being hurt from the daily grind – everyday folks that have to stop working because of chronic pain – arch pain, heel pain or whatever. They are on disability and get put on workers compensation – factory workers, people who are pounding the hard flat surfaces every day."

"Is surgery necessary for knee and hip problems and would they then have to take drugs?"

Dr. John Feulner: "If a joint gets to the point where it is completely destroyed and the patient is in constant pain, then yes, of course surgery is warranted. But with that being said, we stop people from getting surgery routinely. In particular we stop heel spur[253] surgery, which in essence cuts a supporting structure that is pulling on the heel instead of supporting it because the foot and arch has flattened out. We

253 Heel spur: soft, bendable deposits of calcium that are the result of tension and inflammation in the heel

stop them from getting neuroma[254] surgery, bunion surgery, hammertoe surgery, knee or hip surgery or replacement etc...

"Unfortunately, many years of pain, discomfort and drugs that are prescribed to mask the symptoms are what lie on the road that ultimately leads to surgery because it is during this time of imbalance that the joints become destroyed. And then with surgery, one needs to take more drugs to handle the pain and discomfort associated with the surgery itself.

"Then if it doesn't work they have chronic pain from that. Unfortunately in most cases, they don't address the bottom line – the biomechanics – that structural imbalance that destroyed the knees and other joints in the first place. It goes back to good structural alignment."

"What is the technique that you use to correct these imbalances?"

Dr. John Feulner: "If the arch collapses significantly and both feet collapse differently, that creates even more imbalances. When they collapse the same amount it creates a certain amount of imbalance. When they collapse at different degrees that's what starts to affect even more imbalance higher up above the feet.

"We do some passive manipulation such as in house physical therapy, but we generally leave that to the chiropractors and the therapists. What we do mainly is spot the imbalances and handle them with various treatment modalities. The most common approach is to go over what shoes they are wearing currently. We go over each pair and instruct them on what would be a better biomechanically sound shoe for them. Often the changing of their shoe gear handles many problems in itself."

254 Neuroma: a benign tumor composed of nerve tissue creating an inflamed nerve

"And if this is not enough?"

Dr. John Feulner: "The next thing we usually do is to tape or strap the foot with athletic training tape in a very specific way to temporarily hold the foot in the corrective position. This temporary fix allows the patient to experience the benefits of having their foot and body in a corrected position and there is in most cases a corollary in that if the taping works well, then the orthotics will do great. We then offer them the permanent solution, our custom made total contact orthotic arch supports."

"What are the results you get from these treatments?"

Dr. John Feulner: "With people who have shin splints[255], we knock these out in a couple of days. Most people's knee pain, heel pain etc… can be knocked out in hours to days to weeks. We give them such great pain relief they can stop taking their pain medications. Drugs are suddenly unnecessary. In fact, in most cases we offer our patients a 100% satisfaction guarantee."

"Do other Podiatrists operate more with drugs than you do?"

Dr. John Feulner: "Typically speaking, podiatrists are not overly inundated with prescribing drugs, but yes. The first thing that usually happens when someone presents with heel pain, arch pain, a bad knee etc…, and they are in some degree of pain, is for the doctor to give them an injection or some medicine to calm down the inflammation and pain. It is our philosophy that if we stop the torquing or twisting of the joints and the subsequent squashing of the joint spaces, then we will stop the pain. Then there is no need for any

255 Shin splints: painful conditions of the shins caused by inflammation of the surrounding muscles

drugs, for cortisone injections or ultimately for a total knee replacement. Again if we aren't going to correct the structural misalignment, we aren't going to fix the problem or rid the patient of their pain and discomfort."

"Why do the physicians or other practices recommend drugs so readily when it comes to problems with the knee and hip?"

Dr. John Feulner: "We have just become a drug society. People are inundated with medicines and drugs especially around cold and flu season. There are so many commercials now on TV that sell some kind of pill for alleviating this or that. Instead of looking at basic causative actions, factors or alignments, they recommend a drug. When someone has knee pain for example, how about addressing the fact that the joint complex has been compromised? Let's fix some of the cartilage. Let's get some better nutritional stuff in there and not keep on masking the symptoms with drugs."

"How much less drugs do you give in relation to another doctor?"

Dr. John Feulner: "It is rare that we ever give drugs, to any of our patients. Cortisone injections are used as an anti-inflammatory agent but its effects, if used often, can be quite harmful to healthy ligaments and tendons. It deteriorates the collagen, which is the very substance that makes up the ligaments and tendons. We avoid all of that. We rarely if ever give injections or pain medications. I cannot repeat this enough - if we correct the right reason for the imbalance, we eradicate the need for such drugs."

"What about degenerative diseases and the non-steroidal anti-inflammatory drugs people take for them?"

Dr. John Feulner: "There are things like rheumatoid arthritis[256] and psoriatic arthritis.[257] These do degenerate joints and are definitely a reason for total knee and hip replacements but these are by far not the only reasons. People are chronically taking these non-steroidal anti-inflammatory and more severe drugs to handle their discomfort. For example, there is *Motrin,*[258] *Feldene,*[259] *Naprosyn,*[260] *Ibuprofen.*[261] People eat these things like candy. They can adversely affect the liver if the person is on these drugs for an extended amount of time. Doctors tell the patient to get liver tests or "chemistries" to make sure he isn't destroying his liver with long term use."

"What are the effects of those drugs?"

Dr. John Feulner: "Horrible stuff. The patient can get stomach ulcers, chronically upset stomach, liver damage, and hepatic[262] problems especially with long term usage."

"How often have you seen side effects on your patients?"

Dr. John Feulner: "Literally every day we see people at the end of their rope. All too often patients allow their symptoms to be treated with the drugs and then they are sent for some type of physical therapy to strengthen and tone their muscles. When that fails the ultimate cure is a surgical

256 Rheumatoid arthritis: a chronic disease marked by stiffness and inflammation of the joints, weakness, loss of mobility, and deformity

257 Psoriasis: A noncontagious inflammatory skin disease characterized by recurring reddish patches covered with silvery scales

258 Motrin: a trademark name for *ibuprofen*

259 Feldene: a non-steroidal anti-inflammatory drug

260 Naprosyn: a non-steroidal anti-inflammatory drug, is used to relieve the inflammation, swelling, stiffness, and joint pain associated with rheumatoid arthritis, osteoarthritis and other pain related conditions

261 Ibuprofen: a commonly used non-steroidal anti-inflammatory drug used for inflammation and pain

262 Hepatic: acting on or occurring in the liver

one. That's what people ultimately end up going to. Surgery could be called the last side effect. With that being said, there is definitely a time and place for surgery. When joints are destroyed beyond all hope of repair or rehabilitation, a surgical solution is more than appropriate to handle that patient's chronic discomfort. The point here is to not let it get to that point by addressing the underlying structural misalignment that caused the degeneration in the first place and more importantly, do not just cover up the symptoms with drugs.

"What will be the future of this society as you see it?"

Dr. John Feulner: "The future as I see it is nothing but more drugs. Statistically speaking more and more people are taking drugs for everything. Never mind the ridiculousness of the Psychiatric community, making up stuff. How desperate is someone and to what length would they go to have another excuse to give someone else a pill? And this in the face of the recently documented harmful side effects of psych drugs in general. It is really sickening."

"What is the motto for your clinic?"

Dr. John Feulner: "If the patient has any joint or muscle pain, he probably has a structural imbalance. In most every case we can correct that imbalance and alleviate his pain."

7. BEHIND THE CURTAIN: SPORTS MEDICINE AND DRUGS

It was a fantastic event: the 2004 Olympic Games in Greece were really a superlative of all superlatives ... billions of spectators watched on television screens. Many records were broken. Athens hosted 11,099 athletes, the highest ever in history, and there were more women athletes than ever before. There were 202 countries that sent representatives to the games and, from the spectacular opening of the Games to the climatic closing; it was an event that surpassed all other Olympic Games. Indeed it was a year to be remembered.

And doping was of course a topic in the last Olympic winter games during 2006 in Turin, Italy. In a police raid in the quarters of the Austrian team, thirty boxes containing medications and machines for blood tests and blood transfusions were found.

But this is only one side of the medal – of the gold, silver and bronze medal. The other side was, of course, the topic of *drugs*.

The Greeks themselves produced the first scandal. The two sprinters/runners, Konstantinos Kenteris and Ekaterini Thanou – two national heroes, sport-heroes – two fantastic athletes – did not participate in the Olympic games, with all this glamour. Why? Officially it was said they had an accident, but unofficially there was the suspicion that they tried everything to avoid being tested for drugs. But just looking at the body of Konstantinos Kenteris told the professional something: he has legs like the "wheels of a tractor" wrote the SPIEGEL.

USA athletes have the worst reputation, worldwide, when it comes to drugs. The scandal, in relation to the doping laboratory Balco[263] (near San Francisco), is never forgotten: the confessions of runner Kelli White, the positive findings of Torri Edwards.

263 Balco: Bay Area Laboratory Co-Operative that operates as a nutritional supplement lab. Balco allegedly provided baseball stars with illegal performance-enhancing drugs recently.

Tim Montgomery and Regina Jacobs just speak their own language. In 2004, Montgomery was accused of taking performance-enhancing drugs and Jacobs of taking *THG*[264], both also connected to the Balco scandal. And this is not just a recent occurrence. For example, Ben Johnson, who won the gold medal in 1988 for clocking a world record of 9.79 in the 100-meter sprint, was stripped of this medal after he tested positive for a testosterone-treated substance. He attested that this was very common among athletes in all fields.[265] Even then! In 1988!

Meanwhile, there are tests for athletes in existence that are hard to get around. Cheating becomes more and more difficult. Even the designer drug *THG*, and drugs like *EPO*[266] and *Hemopure*[267] can be found today.

Four years earlier, in Sydney, ten athletes were found cheating. In Athena, Greece, at least eleven athletes were caught trying to cheat. But one would be very naïve, believing that this is the true picture. Of course it is just the tip of the iceberg, and when one sees an athlete with bulging muscles, HE KNOWS, even without testing, that there is at least a suspicion that *anabolics* are taken. It is hard to put down exact numbers, one can only guess, but insiders say that one tenth of the professional athletes have at least one time or the other tried anabolics, depending on the discipline. So meanwhile, even the best of the best, when it comes to body-condition, pray to the God, *drug*.

But let us first consider some facts, which include not only athletes but also sportive activities in general.

---

264 THG: a designer steroid *Tetrahydrogestrinone*, derived by some simple chemical modifications of two well known and athletically banned – synthetic steroids, called *trenbolone* and *gestinone.* http://www.usatoday.com/sports/olympics/athens/track/2004-07-17-jacobs-suspension_x.htm

265 "Athletics," *Sports Illustrated*, London, 04 August 1998

266 EPO: *erythropoietin*, a blood-boosting hormone that enhances stamina.

267 *Hemopure* is the brand name for a blood substitute consisting of ultra purified, modified bovine hemoglobin suspended in a salt solution, which contains no red cells. It enhances tissues by increasing oxygen profusion.

FACTS

What is meant by anabolics anyways? Why do the athletes desire them? Anabolic/androgenic steroids are actually what we are talking about when we say anabolics. *Steroids* are drugs that are derived from hormones, and anabolic/androgenic steroids are those belonging to a group of *performance-enhancing* drugs. On the street they are called "juice" or "roids."

You see, there are *useful steroids* that doctors prescribe for one reason or another, such as cortisone for rashes and itching, and estrogen and progesterone for the female reproductive system maintenance, or androgens that maintain the male reproductive system. We are not talking about these, or even their side effects, in this chapter. It is the anabolic/androgenic steroids that we are concerned with here, as you will soon see.

Why do people use them? Athletes use them to gain an advantage over their opponents. Teenagers might use them to develop their bodies so that they gain a better self-image. Doesn't sound too bad, does it? But there is a catch. And before we step into this spider's web, let's have a closer look.

"Anabolic" means growing or building and "androgenic" denotes generating male sexual characteristics. This implies that the steroids taken will aid in the growth of muscles, bones, and skin and also bring about a more masculine body type. Great if one is a guy. They affect aggressiveness and sex drive. The athlete on steroids becomes more aggressive. This gives these athletes an advantage over the athletes not taking steroids, because they enhance strength, endurance and aggressiveness.

Sports are known to be aggressive. Have a look at football, for example. The more aggressive the athlete, the better he will do. Lots of aggressiveness there, great! Except that taking anabolic steroids is an unfair advantage and is deemed cheating by the International Olympics Committee. Taking them has become illegal. And there are hazards in taking them, horrible hazards. But more on that later.

First, what are some of these steroids? Here are some of the most common ones: *Nandrolone*, *Oxancrolone*, *Oxymeholone*, and *Stanozolol*. Other common anabolic steroids taken today are *Anadrol, Oxandrin, Dianabol, Winstrol, Decadurabolin, and Equipoise*. Fancy names, the lot of them. So what do they do? Basically, they are all related to testosterone, a male sex hormone and they help to rebuild tissues and repair tissue injuries. They are muscle builders. But they also do other things that are not desired in the least, as we will find out.

There are many sports in which athletes are interested in building muscles and stamina. Not only in football, as we mentioned earlier, are players suspected of using anabolic steroids. Track and field contestants are also in the game, so to speak. Then there are other sports like wrestling, baseball, and bicycling that require endurance. In the news lately, we find that the NFL[268] is stringently testing their players for steroids and there are severe penalties for testing positive to these drugs. Hooray, we might exclaim.

However, athletes can cover up the existence of steroids in their body by using other drugs. Or they can just stop taking them before the test. So the tests won't show positive in many cases. By the way, it should be noted here that taking them without a prescription from a physician who has not examined that person is illegal.

And it's not only athletes that use anabolic steroids. Just search the Internet for stories of teens who do this not only to excel at the sport they are involved in but also to develop their physique so that they look good (and attract girls).

High school students have been known to secretly take steroids to build their bodies up for some sport to enable them to enter College on a scholarship. This is in addition to improving their appearance and self-image at the risk of developing a dependence on these drugs. Imagine some scrawny, pimple-faced, 15 year old wanting to impress the girl in his class not to mention the jocks in the gym. He is a perfect candidate for a secret stash of these muscle-building crèmes, pills and injections. Along with this, he

268 NFL: National Football League

works out with the machines and he is transformed into the talk of the school. Image booster? We guess so.

This is particularly nasty for the teen as he becomes addicted to the drug (depends on it for his looks and self esteem) and since this is the time of physical development, his natural growth hormones are affected, and his health is at risk. Are we looking at a small percentage? In one study done in 2002 by NIDA,[269] it was seen that 2.4% of eighth graders tried steroids, 3.5% of 10th graders and 4% of twelfth graders. We are not talking about a rare case here. In a school of 600 students, there would be 20 to 24 students taking steroids.

An interview with a local coach who trains pro athletes revealed his own horror story, which we will reveal in a moment. You won't hear many such stories.

WHAT NOBODY DARES TO TALK ABOUT

It is interesting to note here that despite the testing of anabolic steroids going on at the professional level, people are still using them to develop their physique and increase their stamina. But one won't hear about it in the press at the local bodybuilding club. In fact, when one of the authors went down to ask what steroids he would need to take to develop his physique, the owner denied there would be any. Instead, he was told, they use *creatine*[270] and *NO2*,[271] which are legal today. The owner said that no side effects have been mentioned with these two new supplements. But then there are no long-term studies on either of them as well. Who knows what will turn up after extensive use of either? In an interview with a body building coach who no longer uses steroids, the coach mentioned

269 NIDA: National Institute on Drug Abuse

270 *Creatine* is a natural substance found in the body that plays a powerful role in energy metabolism. Taking creatine gives you more energy and allows the taker to exercise longer with out tiring out.

271 NO2 is nitric oxide that triggers the body to an increased blood flow to the muscles. This normally occurs during exercise anyways, but with NO2 this increased blood flow does not stop once exercise has ended. This gives the serious athlete the ability to build muscle around the clock if he so desired.

trying *NO2* and getting the worse headache in his life. Sounds like more work has to be done. We will take a look at other possible side effects later.

In the meantime, the bodybuilding coach states no steroids are being used at the bodybuilding center. And yet, by looking at the physique of the owner pasted on the wall one would tend to wonder if anabolic steroids actually had a part in the development of those tight knots of muscle. Especially when other athletes have said it couldn't be done without anabolic steroids. Makes a person wonder, doesn't it?

And that brings us to that spider web of the side effects that these drugs bring with them.

THE HORRIBLE SIDE EFFECTS OF ANABOLICS/STEROIDS

The body is dependent on the balance of hormones within its system. What happens when someone changes that balance? Testosterone is a male hormone that regulates the male reproductive system. The female also produces a small amount of testosterone, too, but that is in rare amounts. When the female takes anabolic steroids, she takes on male characteristics. These characteristics are irreversible. She will look and sound like a man and remain that way for the rest of her life. What a price to pay!

And take a look at EPO. This modern, popular drug can be bought today over the Internet, reported the Spiegel.[272] It is even available via eBay and here even cheaper than through the normal channels. To avoid getting caught in the controls the athletes just stop taking it a week before the contest.

EPO is a hormone, produced from the extraction of the hormone from the ovaries of the Chinese squirrel, and allegedly increases endurance by pushing the body to produce more red blood cells. It adds oxygen to the blood stream by regulating red-cell production and thus it can improve the athlete's record in a sports event. Imagine a runner improving his speed in a 20-minute

---

272 Der Spiegel 48/2005, p. 147

run by 30 seconds, or four minutes if it is a marathon. This drug is popular for this fact alone by long-distance runners, swimmers and cyclists. But the catch? Bob Hanna, Sports Reporter and Columnist for the *South Coast Today* stated, "An overdose could thicken the blood so much that the heart would not be able to pump it. EPO is believed, according to *Time*,[273] to have caused 25 deaths among Olympic-caliber cyclists in the past 23 years." [274] Now this is what we consider flirting with danger.

EPO is not alone as a dangerous steroid. *Hemopure* tends to cause kidney failure. *THG*, that wonderful designer drug, causes liver damage, heart disease, anxiety, and rage.[275] How wonderful is that?

Note that we haven't even mentioned the side effects of steroids that are injected. Sharing needles or using nonsterile techniques make the user at risk for contracting dangerous infections such as HIV/AIDS, hepatitis B and C, and bacterial endocarditis (inflammation of the thin membrane that lines the interior of the heart).[276]

Other steroids cause tumors of the liver or liver cancer, and even affect blood sugar levels. Then there is acne and moodiness and high blood pressure.

Often, athletes use more than one kind of steroid at a time. This is called 'stacking' and supposedly allows the user to get bigger faster. Or they will pyramid their doses in six- to twelve-week cycles meaning that they start out with low doses and increase the dose gradually. In either case, overdosing is possible, which brings about more side effects and more harm to the body.

The local coach's horror story we mentioned earlier, illustrates well what we are talking about. In 1986, he was on a winning streak. The steroids he had used were serving him well and he was in the state championship. When he first started taking them,

---

273 Sullivan/Song, "Are Drugs Winning The Games?" *Time Magazine,* 11 September 2000

274 http://www.southcoasttoday.com/daily/09-00/09-22-00/c01sp094.htm

275 http://www.sportsline.com/olympics/story/6786641

276 Alan Leshner, Ph.D., "Anabolic Steroid," *NIDA*, 2004 http://www.nida.nih.gov/PDF/RRSteroids.pdf

he gained 33 pounds in muscle in the first 6 weeks. What could possibly go wrong? Everything. At first there were the side effects of moodiness, bad skin, high blood pressure and liver problems. But then came the final horror. He had built up his muscles too fast and during the championship blew out his legs. Muscles, tendons, and ligaments were all torn out.

As a result he spent four months in a hospital bed undergoing a complete restoration of his legs. This involved operations using pins and plates and resulting in scars. In fact, he was told he might never walk again. What a nightmare for a promising champion! He swore off the steroids and worked hard at rehabilitating his legs and after nine months he was finally able to walk. Benefits? There were none.

Even *Creatine* has its side effects, even though *authorities* state that there are none. In *Mosby's Handbook of Herbs and Natural Supplements*, author Linda Skidmore-Rath states that Creatine can cause nausea, anorexia, bloating, weight gain, diarrhea, dehydration, and cramping (with high doses).[277] All this for less than 1 hour of workability during the performance of exercise or sports. Only 1 hour of benefits for all those side effects. Imagine that!

People who have renal or cardiac disease are even advised not to take Creatine.

THE HISTORY OF DOPING

The history of doping starts at the beginning of last century. From the beginning, *alcohol*, *cocaine* and *heroin* were used. And yes, even *strychnine*.

Pain was suppressed this way. The side effects were delirium, alcohol dependency, cramps, breathing difficulties, and heart-rhythm problems.

In the Fifties and Sixties, *Amphetamines* joined the club. The side effects of these were trembling, heart-rhythm problems and heart attacks, aggressiveness and psychological problems.

277 Linda Skidmore-Rath, *Mosby's Handbook of Herbs and Natural Supplements, 2nd Edition,* (St. Louis, Missouri: Mosby Inc, 2004,) pp. 325 – 326

In the Seventies and Eighties, *steroids* and *cortisone* were used for muscle building. *Steroids* caused impotence, damage to the liver, possible heart attacks, skin problems, and explosive emotions. *Cortisone* is bad for the skin as well. It can lower blood pressure and body temperature.

In the Nineties and up to today, *Epo* is the new "miracle drug," plus the treatment with one's own blood. The side effects of *Epo* are viscous and sticky blood, which causes the blood to have difficulty flowing, and the heart to stop. Who committed the doping? Well, the athletes themselves were responsible, but one should not forget that they were influenced and "advised" by doctors. And behind them stood the pharmaceutical industry.

Let's look at just one area in which many athletes admitted to doping and were disqualified: cycling. In cycling, a lot of scandals are well documented. Since 1966, only three winners out of twenty-two in the Tour de France did not take dope (or at least were not accused of doping). Everything has been used: *Amphetamines, Corticoid, Anabolic* substances, growth hormones and, repeatedly, *Epo*.

Today *Epo* is really the "in" thing to do. *Epo* is short for *Erythropoietin*, which enhances the production of the red blood cells and brings more oxygen into the blood. Pills were eaten and substances injected; cyclers doped themselves left, right and center.

Here are just a few of the scandals: Fausto Coppi (Italy), who won the Tour de France twice, admitted he had taken Amphetamines. (1950s). Tom Simpson (Great Britain) who admitted the same "fault" died during the Tour de France (1967). Rudi Altig (Germany) admitted the same "mistake" (1969). Eddy MerckX (Belgium) also took Amphetamines (1969). Walter Godefroot (Belgium) took Ritalin (1974). Alex Zülle (Switzerland) took *Epo* (1998). Christian Henn (Germany) "helped" himself with Testosterone (1999). Johan Museeuw (Belgium) took *Epo* (2004). Tyler Hamilton (USA) doped himself with blood. (2004). David Millar (Great Britain) took *Epo* (2004). Lance Armstrong (USA) took *Epo* (2005). Floyd Landis

(USA) had artificially induced Testosterone in his body when he was tested, but he fought against the test (2006). (Each case is documented well by the SPIEGEL, 2007.)

All those superstars! All those megastars!

Of course, there are techniques already in existence on how to "beat" the controls. One of these tricks was for the cycler to "handle" his urine before the test (to find out if the athlete took forbidden drugs or not took place). First the urinary bladder is narcotized or deadened with *Xylocain*, to deaden the pain. Then a little pipe is induced about 20 cm deep into the urinary bladder. On the end of this little pipe is a tiny ball that helps to find out when the inner muscle is reached. One pricks through and the urinary bladder is emptied. The old urine of the cycler is discarded. Then the urinary bladder is cleaned up with a special solution. The third step consists of emptying the urinary bladder once again. Then, step No. 4, another person's fresh, clean urine is put into the sports hero's urinary bladder. The test can then take place… and nothing will be found. (Source: The book of Jef D`Hont, Memoires, 2007)

PRESENT TIME DOPING

In addition, the pharmaceutical industry conducts further research continuously into *Epo*, and creates new *Epo* products. Meanwhile, more than ten different *Epo*-pharmaceuticals exist, which cannot be tested by the controllers. *Epo-mimetika* "mimic" the *Epo* effects. Sometimes little chemical changes help to fool the controllers, so nothing can be found in the urine or in the blood. What also "works" is to corrupt the controllers. Products from Russia and China are sold on the black market. More than ten billion dollars each year is profited with *Epo*.

However, cycling is just one example. One can find other examples in baseball, boxing, football, heavy-weight lifting, skiing, tennis, sprinting, swimming, wrestling and even golf. The most obvious is body building. Body building is contaminated with drugs – one just has to look at all those artificial muscles, and know without further investigation. Anabolica is the talk of the day in fitness studios. Insiders talk about structures similar to the illegal drug market. Four out of ten professional athletes enrolled in fitness centers take drugs. And a higher percentage of them are younger in age.

But the consequences are horrible. High blood pressure, hair growing in the wrong place, loss of hair on the head, shrinking testicles, men developing breasts, aggressions, organ damage, and even death … these are just some of the side effects. Quite often youngsters finance their consumption of anabolica by dealing. Some travel to Spain, Greece, Cyprus or Turkey. Weird Internet providers offer anabolica as well. But anabolica is often just the beginning stage for street drugs like Ecstasy or even cocaine.

THE KICKER

Now people don't even know that nutritional supplements can have hormones today. They don't know that exercise, a very good thing usually, can make things worse. They don't know that anabolic/steroids can interact with other medication. They don't know what they are REALLY up against. Taking anabolic steroids with many common medicines such as *acetaminophen* (*Tylenol*), estrogens, anti-thyroid agents, birth control pills, and many others increase the chance of liver damage. Taking steroids with anticoagulants taken by mouth increase the effect of these medicines and can cause excessive bleeding.

Steroids worsen conditions of heart or blood vessel disease by increasing blood cholesterol levels. They worsen kidney disease, liver disease, and prostate cancer. Steroids worsen even diabetes as it decreases blood sugar levels. How does the athlete know that he does not have any of these conditions before taking the steroids?

THE FUTURE

In fact, the topic *sports and drugs* is a never-ending subject. We gave only a few data here, and not to the true extent, because there are too many unknowns, too many secrets here. Probably more than anyone can tell.

However, what is not known are the mental side effects of anabolic/steroids.

We already heard that increased aggressiveness might be the case. In other words, one has to look at the emotional side of those side effects. Yes, one can turn a woman into a man and a man can develop female breasts, and man and woman can die from anabolic/steroids. But that is only part of the picture.

Imagine that someone programs himself to be continuously aggressive – continuously half in anger – continuously ready to attack.

He changes his *emotions* entirely that way. While aggressiveness and even anger sometimes may have some value from time to time, it's certainly nuts to act covertly or overtly angry and aggressive all the time. In fact he turns himself into another personality that way.

Yes, he turns himself into a drug-personality with characteristics and traits he never had before. Perhaps he becomes like an aggressive dog with an uncontrollable urge to attack.

His whole viewpoint changes and, in general, his perspective to life changes. Manipulating himself into an emotionally fixated state, he will make different decisions and his life will be different. It will be horrible, because in the end he will not be the personality he really is. Instead he will be an artificial drug personality with artificial emotions and a self-imposed, self-manipulated view of life.

He could have increased problems with his environment – who knows?

The athletes, in taking drugs, turn themselves into another personality just like any other drug-consumer.

Perhaps in the future, we will have different types of drug-personalities: the aggressive type, the silent type, the apathetic-lethargic type, the hallucinatory type, the obedient-type, etc.

We will lose our identity, our true self.

The "winner" will again be the pharmaceutical industry.

The pharmaceutical industry will sell and sell and sell; they will innocently say they don't like the illegal use of anabolic steroids, but they will take the dollars earned from it.

The pharmaceutical industry will turn even the best of us (and the athletes belong to the best) into emotionally changed personalities – into emotional robots.

One could write a whole book on this fact alone: what medical drugs are doing to musicians, to actors and to Hollywood in general. The point is: all those people, including the Yuppies and the super successful, are *target markets* for the pharmaceutical industry. And all that this industry has to do is to tell those ambitious people, that drugs will:

- make you more successful
- make you better looking (think of all those breast implants for which again drugs are used at least for anesthetic reasons)
- make you smarter and more intelligent
- help you get a better job, etc.

You see the potential marketing of those *success-drugs*? Partially that is already the case; some drugs promise parents that their children can learn better, some promise beauty (a whole industry) but there will be even more sophisticated drugs in the future, attached to the topic *success*, for which athletes are only one example. Money, money, money, wherever we look.

We can see then that, for the pharmaceutical industry, side effects are not really important. The legal damage has to be handled, yes, but basically the goal of every pharmaceutical company is to sell more drugs. That is the objective.

With this statement we are now facing the actual scandal, after the following interview.

DR. GREG OLSON: "HANDS ON HOLISTIC HEALTH CARE."

Two segments of the population who direly need chiropractic help to increase their health potential are the athletes and the indigents.[278]

The athlete's endeavor is to overcome their opponent(s) in order to win and thus survive. To do so in today's competitive world seems to dictate that one takes steroids to improve one's endurance and strength. These same steroids that are said to improve the musculature and stamina of the athlete are a hidden Trojan horse in that they insidiously damage the body in many ways unknown to the imbiber. For the past several years, and more so recently, athletes have been known to be taking steroids even though various testing has been occurring to expose the user. However, steroid use has been widespread ever since the early 20th century. Anabolic steroids were developed in the 1930s and began to be used widely by weight lifters and body builders.

There has been a recent effort on the part of World Anti-Doping Agency (WADA) to impose drug testing standards on American professional sports leagues, but how successful these tests are appears yet to be known. For example, it has been stated in the magazine *Men's Fitness* that "of the four major American team sports, only the NFL[279] has what appears to be a serious drug-testing program." It goes on to say that even though "most of its athletes are tested multiple times throughout the year … the average size of the offensive linemen on one NFL team increased 19% – from 260 to 309 pounds, according to *Sports Illustrated*."[280] So even this drug-testing program is up to question.

There are still many athletes that are flunking the tests for steroids and suffering the consequences of that and even the testing procedures are deemed inadequate.

278 Indigents: low-income people

279 NFL: National Football League

280 "The Juice is Loose," *Men's Fitness,* March 07, 2005

The other group of people needing chiropractic care is the indigent. The indigent sits on the dole[281] because he is unable to work due to some chronic misalignment of his skeletal or muscular system. Surveyed, the poor state that they would rather work than be on the welfare system, but the state of their body demands otherwise from them.

Dr. Greg Olson has dedicated his time and expertise in the chiropractic field to treat these two groups of people as well as work with others that come to see him. He cares about the productive state of the poor and the future health of the athlete. As a result, he is very familiar with the scene and is able to give us additional insight.

"First we would like to know a bit about your background. What is your educational experience?"

Dr. Greg Olson: "I have an Associate degree in Liberal Arts[282] from the Golden Valley Lutheran College in 1980, a Bachelors degree in Philosophy from the University of Minnesota in 1981. Then I received my Graduate from Northwestern College of Chiropractic in Aug of 1995 and became a bona fide Certified Chiropractic Neurologist[283] in 1991."

"How many patients have you treated up to today?"

Dr. Greg Olson: "In the past 20 years I have treated approximately 10,000 patients."

"Have you received any honors, awards or certificates?"

281 Dole: welfare

282 Liberal Arts: academic disciplines, such as languages, literature, history, philosophy, mathematics, and science, that provides information of general cultural concern

283 Chiropractic Neurology: the study of how nerves work and how chiropractic relates to the function of the nervous system

Dr. Greg Olson: "Yes. In the past, I was the president of Metro West Chiropractic Association of Minnesota. Currently, I am the chiropractor secretary of the USA Judo Sports Medicine Sub committee and the chiropractor on the executive committee."

"Is it true that you concentrate on the poor people of the community?"

Dr. Greg Olson: "We do work a lot with the poorer folk in town. If these people are brought back to good health and a better life style, it puts them back into the work force. This helps everyone all around. We also treat athletes as well – particularly professional boxers. That is the best joy of my life."

"Why concentrate on the poor and the athletes?"

Dr. Greg Olson: "With the impoverished there is the irony in that when we have people who can't work, it is due to a back or knee condition. Fix these things and they would go back to work and their families would be off welfare."

"Does medical assistance cover Chiropractic care?"

Dr. Greg Olson: "The way that the health system is designed, the first thing to drop out is chiropractic. And yet this is what the patient needs in order to go back to work. If he is given an option of going back to work or continuing on with a medical condition, he would choose going to work and becoming productive in society again. Modern medicines don't offer this kind of medical help when it comes to problems with the body being out of alignment."

"You say you also specialize in treating athletes. Do you like sports?"

Dr. Greg Olson: "I have been involved in sports myself quite a bit having wrestled through high school and college. I also have a black belt in Judo."

"How many athletes have you treated?"

Dr. Greg Olson: "I have treated literally hundreds of athletes."

"What about the use of drugs by athletes? What is your opinion on that subject?"

Dr. Greg Olson: "I see that there are several things going on here and the most dangerous one is that they are taken illegally. Steroids are prevalent in sports even with the testing and restrictions on their dispensation."

"What percentage would you say take steroids?"

Dr. Greg Olson: "My wild guess is that about half of all athletes are on steroids. Eight years ago I was working with a sports writer who made the comment that there were more steroids in baseball than any other sport."

"Why is that?"

Dr. Greg Olson: "Baseball is a short burst sport. The player needs quick energy for a short period of time during the game. This is how the drugs work. Other short burst sports are basketball and hockey and there are a lot of athletes in these sports also that use steroids."

"What percentage of the athletes in Olympic Games take steroids, would you say?"

Dr. Greg Olson: "Probably one third does. Male athletes take more than female athletes, but I have seen women with muscles too. You can tell they are taking a variation of a male hormone called *dihydrotestosterone*[284] by the balding effect it creates. Taking dihydrotestosterone, by the way, has other side effects such as severe acne, causing permanent scarring. In men, it causes the enlarging of the prostate and in some cases feminization. This is where the male takes on more feminine qualities such as enlarged breasts, fatty deposits and extremely soft muscles."

"How does it affect females?"

Dr. Greg Olson: "Females may become more masculine in that they develop facial hair, deepened voices, irregular menstrual cycles and rougher shin texture. In many cases, the athlete needs additional drugs to counteract these side effects so it becomes a dwindling spiral in the long run."

"Can we assume, then, that athletes with extraordinarily huge muscles are taking steroids?"

Dr. Greg Olson: "Not always. Today's nutrition, in relation to training, is so vast compared to 30 years ago that some people are just predisposed to being critically muscular. That wouldn't have been the case around 30 years ago. For example, there are many supplements on the market these days that help to build up muscle and there is a lot more data available today on the various foods and how they affect the body."

---

284 Dihydrotestosterone: an androgen (a steroid hormone that controls the development and maintenance of masculine characteristics) derived from testosterone and having tumor-suppressing capabilities useful in the treatment of certain breast cancers

"What is that nutrition today?"

Dr. Greg Olson: "To start with, there are various mineral and vitamin supplements available today designed especially for athletes. Creatine[285] supplements are known to increase the muscle mass and increase weight which is ideal for the athlete. Amino acids[286] are often needed if not enough is ingested in the diet since otherwise the body will tend to break down muscle to obtain it. The athlete wants to build up the muscle not break it down.

"He is also encouraged to eat a diet high in carbohydrates so that during sports he has the energy to burn. On the market today is a vast array of carbohydrates to choose from, all of which are easily accessible. And of course there are many combinations of herbal remedies that give energy bursts."

"What about the idea of free radicals[287] affecting the body of the athlete?"

Dr. Greg Olson: "Body functions and external influences such as pollution create free radicals which may harm the cells of the body, thus causing illness and possibly cancer. The athlete is definitely concerned about these."

"Where do these free radicals come from?"

Dr. Greg Olson: "Smoking causes free radicals. So does alcohol, prescription drugs, sun bathing and the additives

---

285 Creatine is a substance naturally produced by the body that helps to improve muscle performance during exercise. It is naturally found in meat and fish but is also made by the liver, pancreas, and kidneys within the body itself.

286 Amino acids combine to form proteins and are necessary to build muscles.

287 Free radicals are atoms or group of atoms that has at least one unpaired electron and is therefore unstable and highly reactive. In animal tissues, free radicals can damage cells and are believed to accelerate the progression of cancer, cardiovascular disease and age-related diseases.

and chemicals added to the food we eat. Even the air that we breathe contains free radicals."

"How do they cause the body damage?"

Dr. Greg Olson: "Since free radicals are chemically active atoms or molecular fragments having an excess or deficient number of electrons, they scavenge the body to grab or donate electrons and this damages cells, proteins and DNA.[288] This process is the same one that causes iron to rust and apples to turn brown. Free radicals bring about oxidation in the blood and this in turn opens the door to disease. They also damage healthy cells and weaken the immune system."

"How can the athlete or even the average person prevent the damage done by free radicals?"

Dr. Greg Olson: "There are various antioxidants available that will interact with them and deem them useless. Antioxidants basically give or take the extra electron and neutralize the radical so that it cannot take or give electrons from the healthy cells."

"What are some of these antioxidants?"

Dr. Greg Olson: "Antioxidants are found naturally in the body and in the fruits and vegetables that we eat. The vitamins that are known antioxidants are vitamin A, C and E. If the person is not getting enough antioxidants from the food he eats, there are also antioxidants manufactured on the market that are beneficial such as hawthorn berry, selenium, green tea extract, blue green algae and beta carotene just to name a few."

---

288 DNA: the basic material within the living cell that transmits the hereditary pattern

"What are the favorite medications that athletes currently take?"

Dr. Greg Olson: "They are *deca durabolin*, *winstrol*, *anabar*, *testosterone* and *dianabol* which are all names of various anabolic steroids."[289]

"What side effects do these have?"

Dr. Greg Olson: "What happens when someone takes steroids is that the body thinks it has this normal amount of testosterone and the testicles receive the order not to produce as much testosterone. They start to shut down and the rest of the system shuts down along that axis. The adrenal hormones shut down as well as other hormone systems including the thyroid. The body is made to believe it has all this hormone and when he goes off of it, he is deficient. The body does not make any on its own anymore."

"Does this effect procreation?"

Dr. Greg Olson: "Oh, yes. It may not be impossible, but it is much more difficult."

"What other effects are there?"

Dr. Greg Olson: "As with other toxins, the body needs to get rid of the extra steroids and this is through the liver. Steroids are very toxic and hard on the liver so one gets liver cancer, which is common. Also, since the steroids cause muscles to grow, the heart muscle also grows resulting in an enlarged heart. Body builders end up with cardiac problems in many cases."

---

289 Anabolic steroids: a group of synthetic hormones developed from testosterone that promotes the storage of protein and the development of muscle tissue

"You mentioned balding earlier. Do steroids cause that?"

Dr. Greg Olson: "Testosterone does tend to make hair fall out. The use of the steroid causes the immune system to react to the hair follicles as foreign bodies. The body destroys them thus leading to baldness."

"How about the emotional effect of steroids on people?"

Dr. Greg Olson: "Testosterone and similar drugs give the person taking them a bad attitude, making them aggressive. They can then go into, what is called, a *'roid rage* which is an irrational response to their environment involving extreme anger."

"Would you say they turn people into emotional robots?"

Dr. Greg Olson: "Definitely! The user acts aggressively in every situation even if it is illogical. This aggression may be useful in sports but does not fit the scene in normal everyday living."

"What would you say are the worst case scenarios with side effects?"

Dr. Greg Olson: "People are known to commit murder while in a 'roid rage. One well-known example of this is Sally McNeal.[290] She killed her significant other with a 12-gauge shot gun, thinking he was having an affair. She was on steroids at the time."

"Does severe body damage occur with the intake of these drugs?"

290 Sally McNeal: one of the most popular and loved female bodybuilders who competed in wrestling

Dr. Greg Olson: "Severe damage is probably very small, but the risk of that is great. Body builders take 100 times the recommended medical dosage and they have lots of things wrong with them physically. Their hormonal system is out of whack and the various organs do not function normally."

"With the nutrition so bad these days, does this cause any bad interaction with the steroid medication?"

Dr. Greg Olson: "Absolutely! Protein sources that are used such as chicken, turkey, beef and pork, have already been injected with various chemicals such as steroids and antibiotics, etc. Since the person on steroids is already at the highest level that the body can barely compensate for, the food with its additives add to the toxicity rather than help them deal with it."

"In your practice have you handled any special cases with horrible side effects?"

Dr. Greg Olson: "Yes, I had a regional professional whose endocrine system shut down on him. All his hair fell out literally overnight and he started having liver problems. Sex was impossible. He spent seven years of endocrinological treatment trying to get life back in balance. He was on very high doses of steroids and needed ongoing endocrinological care."

"Any others?"

Dr. Greg Olson: "I had a patient using steroids who slapped a customer at his work hard enough to break his jaw. This was the typical 'roid rage at work here. He is now in jail. Athletes who take steroids act like any other drug addict. They are no longer a team member. On steroids, they are very agitated – bouncing off the wall – and they have very odd inappropriate behavior, acting more like beast than man."

"Nowadays, there are ongoing tests that the athletes have to undergo. Are there techniques to cover up steroids?"

Dr. Greg Olson: "There are two ways the athlete tries to do this. One, he could replace the urine sample with another urine sample. This is difficult because the taking of the urine sample is chaperoned by a guard who also accompanies the sample to the testing agency. The second way is to discontinue taking the drug within a certain time. Although he would still have the effect of the drug, the chemistry will be that of someone at the higher end of normal as opposed to abnormal. So he would have big muscles, but he wouldn't have a high testosterone level."

"Is there a struggle then between the two factions of finding new cover-ups and finding ways to detect the new cover-up?"

Dr. Greg Olson: "Absolutely correct. It's an ongoing war pretty much and becomes a contest for the athlete to find a cover-up without being detected. Chiropractically speaking, it's bad for the body in the long run. Either the athlete would need to stop taking it or limit it."

"Who are the drug pushers in this case? Is it the trainers or the doctors? Or is it the pharmaceutical companies?"

Dr. Greg Olson: "There are some doctors who will prescribe them but not many as the drugs are highly protected and the DEA[291] watches like a hawk. And some of the trainers and

291 DEA: Drug Enforcement Administration

other athletes are able to get their hands on it and provide the drugs. But one can easily buy them over the Internet or go to Mexico and buy them legally there."

"Why Mexico?"

Dr. Greg Olson: "They don't have any legal restrictions on it. Even young people are able to get a hold of these drugs."

"Do young athletes have a problem with steroid use also?"

Dr. Greg Olson: "Oh yes. Just recently an article appeared in the *USA Today* that reported a high school football team was having trouble with two of its athletes taking steroids. It went on to say that national surveys showed that 3% to 3.5% of high school students have used steroids. In California alone the estimated number of high school athletes taking steroids is about 20,000."

"Doesn't this have a bad effect on the young person as he matures?"

Dr. Greg Olson: "Yes. For one thing steroids are addictive and often teens will turn to other drugs. It also can cause sterility, stunted growth and masculinity in girls. All of these are undesirable as the youth gets older."

"Are there any non-steroid drugs that create a problem physically for the athlete?"

Dr. Greg Olson: "There are several over-the-counter medications that create problems. For example, take *ibuprofen* and *aspirin*. Combat athletes do get beat up a lot and so take these medications to relieve the inflammation and pain. At first they seem like a Godsend, but in the long run several problems crop up. Not only are they are hard on the stomach, but they increase the fragility of the capillaries and the body bruises more easily. They also create kidney and liver problems. There are natural pain remedies, though, and calcium and magnesium are great for the relief of sore muscles."

"How do you help the patient who has been on steroids?"

Dr. Greg Olson: "The first thing is to get them to stop taking the drugs and get them onto proper nutrition. Then we can also treat them with chiropractic to balance their body's muscle and skeletal system. It's always important to unblock the nerve channels and improve the flow of health to all parts of the body."

"Do you have any motto that you follow?"

Dr. Greg Olson: "Yes. Hands on Holistic health care."

8. OTHER PROFITABLE TARGET MARKETS

With this strategy to define precise target markets, we suddenly start to understand. Unexpectedly all the little bits and pieces of the puzzle fall into place. And yet there is another target market, which is so secretive, and profitable that even the very investigative journalists have never looked at it. We are talking about the hottest of all subjects; we are talking about the military.

Soldiers are a wonderful target market, because here exists all the money in the world. There are billions of tax-dollars, which have to be spent! Let's just look at the Iraq war. Just one little war. Let's not talk about the weapon dealers, which made an unbelievable amount of money with this war. (2.1 billion dollars were spent by the USA every day.) Let's not talk about the oil business and connections of some high politicians to the oil, which has been documented so well by CIA officer Robert Baer. Let's not talk about the "reconstruction" firms that earned billions and the real estate deals that are fantastic in every war. Let's not talk about the "connections" of some high USA politicians to the pharmaceutical industry. But let us talk about the *profits* Big Pharma made.

Oh what a wonderful paradise!

Because of the potential terrorism and bio terrorism threat, first the population was put systematically into panic. Vaccinations suddenly were the talk of the day. The soldiers had to be vaccinated. *Our soldiers* had to be safe.

Let's quickly remember, that vaccinations are the biggest business one can imagine. Since vaccination had some good effects in the past without a doubt, vaccinations were looked at with respect. So fairly early on, big Pharma concentrated on those gigantic markets. Let's look back. In 1994, 3 billion a year was already spent for vaccinations.[292] Who earned the big bucks? Well, our old well-known "friends," *Merck, Smith-Kline-Beecham but*

292 Tim O'Shea, p. 46

also Pasteur-Merieux-Connaught, and Biocine-Sclavo and Wyeth-Lederle.

AlphaVax, a large vaccine research company in the USA, can use public funds to develop new vaccinations. The market grew and grew. Up to 4 billion dollars, up to 5 billion dollars at the moment 10% each year.

Twelve billion injections are given per year to keep the population of earth safe, says WHO, The World Health Organization. Boy, are we talking about big business here, which insofar is very attractive as it is a growing market! Every new disease brings about further vaccinations.

Unknown is the fact, that the human body, treated with too many vaccinations, can collapse and be sicker in the end. Not known is the fact that in some vaccinations lethal mercury is present. Not known is the fact that there are many side effects possible from vaccination. Not known is the fact that some vaccinations can kill people. But what is known is the fact that vaccinations allegedly help against diseases.

Now back to our soldiers. Let's even go back to the first Iraq war. Desert Storm happened in 1991. Six hundred and ninety-six soldiers received several vaccinations. And now comes the real surprise. "During the following three years some 80 thousand of those troops checked into VA hospitals with serious neurological and degenerative diseases for which they had no previous history. Collectively, these mysterious new illnesses came to be known as the Gulf War Syndrome." (O'Shea, pg. 140) Investigations followed, and investigation of investigations. Senators and committees came into view. The result? Unproven chemicals and untested vaccines were given to those soldiers. Well, what a surprise! The military has a history being used for dangerous experiments. But let us stay on Iraq war number one. Some side effects of just one vaccination were these: memory loss, blurred vision, vomiting, urinary irregularities, abdominal cramps, asthma, respiratory disease, and intestinal blockage.

Some soldiers were vaccinated against anthrax. Anthrax once was the talk of the day. An unapproved vaccine to protect against this animal disease was injected to those soldiers; 150 thousand soldiers received anthrax vaccine without data on humans in existence. This vaccine had only been tested on cattle and sheep. It was found that government contracts were given to former joint chief, who held attractive stocks of the founded vaccine company. (O`Shea, pg. 143)

The military personnel had no choice but to receive these dangerous vaccinations. In the end the report stated, there were 43% that had side effects from the vaccinations during the Gulf War. Repeat: 43%.

The black book about military vaccination has not yet been written. Data on the first Iraq war exists; the 2nd Iraq war is not even evaluated yet. But this much is known, and again vaccinations were the talk of the day. And soldiers face demotion, fines and even dismissal when they don't obey. Despite the horrific findings, anthrax vaccine in 2003 was reinstated. Big Pharma started to recommend those vaccinations for the non-military personnel as well. Boy, talk about business! The new war against the Iraqis again brought billions and billions of dollars, just by vaccinations. And the story continues. Who paid for the *medical expenses* during the war? The medical expenses are unbelievable high, because, in a war, people are continuously crippled, wounded, and get sick. Who pays and who *earns*?

After the war, the story even gets better. Soldiers do have problems. Medical problems, body problems, and *psychological* problems. Who takes care just of these psychological problems? Well psychiatrists of course.

What is the diagnosis of those "psychological" problems? Oh, simple. Soldiers suffering after a war have PTSD. PTSD? Post Traumatic Stress Disorder. Take this word apart, which sounds so impressive and it doesn't say anything. It says there are psychic problems after wars. How many soldiers had PTSD after the second Iraq war? Admittedly 17%, but half of it, state insiders, just don't talk about it, because they are ashamed. They don't want to disqualify themselves; they want to appear strong because a soldier is strong, isn't he? A soldier is a tough guy, not somebody with PTSD.

Who handles this Post Traumatic Stress Disorder? Well the psychiatrists of course. How? With pills naturally. And here we are again. Pills, pills, pills; profit, profit, profit! We play the name game. We have a problem, we give it a good sounding impressive name and invent a pill for it, or we use some existing pills. A third time, the pharmaceutical industry makes the big buck. First time: vaccinations. Second time: during the war by medical support. A third time: after the war.

War is unbelievably, financially interesting for Big Pharma.

And that is not even all; all those newly detected diseases are future target markets. New vaccines are developed right now and are in the pipeline. Vaccines against Herpes simplex, Hepatitis C, Gonorrhea, Asthma, Sars, cancer, tobacco addiction, allergies, and AIDS of course. Billions and billions of dollars are here to be earned in the future. Inside the laboratories, new vaccines are tested against each and every thing because there is no bigger business. Forgotten is the fact that this is the wrong path to vibrant heath; that it weakens the immune system in the long run; and forgotten are the horrible side effects. It's big business.

So soldiers are target markets, wonderful ones, because they seldom fight back, they are trained to obey. Each new disease is a wonderful new target market. The old diseases (aids and cancer) are at any rate, if not only for the vaccination professionals.

Understand this: it is unbelievably good news for the pharmaceutical industry, if there is a new threat, a new disease.

Mass panic sells.

The chaos merchant *loves* bad news and new threats. TV, radio, magazines and newspaper help sell Big Pharma, willy nilly.

The more diseases there are, the better. Look what amount of money went into Aids alone. Do you see the game?

The following can be predicted very easily: with new health threats, new diseases are on the horizon. Our planet is so small and interconnected that a disease in China can be exploited in the USA.

Side effects? Please don't talk about that. Don't destroy our nice little game! And look, those diseases are *real*. See all those dead bodies over there?

Even in dentistry, we find drugs such as lidocaine with epinephrine, anti-coagulants to stop bleeding, and nitrous oxide. And of course there are many side effects here as well. Are these drugs absolutely necessary? Some patients don't really need them, but dentists prefer to administer them just in case. Makes life a bit easier for all concerned. If we negate the side effects, that is. Nevertheless, the side effects are present and cannot be ignored. Even amalgam/mercury fillings have vast side effects, as is currently becoming more and more apparent. This is too highly documented to gloss over.

Here are target markets, wonderful new targets markets. And the marketing is done by the media worldwide, not realizing that even a picture can cause feelings of fears and weaken the immune system. A dangerous environment can make people sick.

So we enter a new world of target markets. Is that all? On no, no! Just look around. Look at those animals. My God, animals!

Did you know that animals could be used wonderfully as a new target market? Dogs and cats have to get pills to "protect" them against disease. Animals are one of the biggest target markets today, growing with an enormous speed.

What are we talking about here? Are we speaking about kittens, birds, lambs, monkeys, ferrets and mice being used for unnecessary cruel pharmaceutical experiments? No. Are we referring to the ten thousand rabbits that are killed to provide a doctor title to someone because he has to "prove," by conducting a large experiment, that animals die if one treats them with a special substance? No. That some doctors cause bleeding surgical wounds, infected brains in animals, or slice their eyes out with scalpels, to prove whatever?

No. Do we talk about doping; that horses get doped today so that they show higher performances on the racetrack?[293] No.

We are speaking about the over-medication and systematic medication of our beloved dogs and cats. Steroids and all sorts of medication are given more and more. Meanwhile there even exists *Prozac* for our animals. Why? A big, new, target market.

And so we could go on and on. Goldmines wherever the eye looks. And yet, we haven't talked about the real scandal.

293 In the last Olympic games (Athena), from 40 horses, four were found to have substances in their urine, not permitted by the rules, stimulating substances, hormone-like substances. See Olaf Stampf, Spiegel 46/2004, pf. 174.

9. THE ACTUAL SCANDAL

After all this information, one might think that he cannot add any further facts. And yet we have only a rough picture of the situation. By the end of this chapter, the *actual* scandal is revealed, which isn't even vaguely seen by most of us. But first, let us reiterate what we already know up to this point, before we come to the true scandal and the true proportion of the drug society.

The fact is we do have a fantastic amount of side effects when it comes to drugs. Just while writing this book, the authors innocently watched the news and heard that *Merck* took *Vioxx*, a medication we mentioned in the beginning of this book as supposedly having an anti-inflammatory effect, off the market. The CEO stated on TV (September 30, 2004) that the withdrawal of this drug happened, not because the company itself wasn't forced to do so, but by the decision of Merck-Management. How noble! The journalist stated (Jim Lehrer-channel) that over 2 billion dollars have been earned (per year) with *Vioxx*, and that without warning a great number of people taking *Vioxx* had heart attacks and strokes. An expert spoke about the huge increase of cardiovascular problems caused by *Vioxx*, and stated that probably thousands and thousands of people died because of this drug. When the journalist innocently asked how that could happen and why *Vioxx* wasn't tested more carefully, the expert's answer was that some drugs get tested only six months and some only six weeks. Some drugs are, in other words, NOT tested when it comes to *long-term* side effects. However, the company still earned *billions*.

So, when it comes to these mysterious *side effects* or ADR (Adverse Drugs Reactions), *years* sometimes go by until the true side effects come to our attention. People on drugs, on medical drugs, on prescriptions drugs, or on over-the-counter drugs, must know that a *huge* risk goes along with this. This risk is probably far greater than normally envisioned. Even the USA Food and Drug

Administration admit: "Safe (drugs) does not mean harmless."[294] Drugs are usually only tested on a few thousand subjects; serious adverse effects will perhaps come to light, perhaps not, but long-term side effects can never be seen in the beginning. In theory, the FDA is the watchdog-committee when it comes to drugs. But something like 10,000 drugs will be evaluated by this agency.

How will that be accomplished?

Let's take a quick look at some of these scandals:

- The drug *Prepulsid* can cause death, and has caused death since 1993.
- *Sandimmune:* 46% of the people being treated with *Sandimmune* for psoriasis had to stop because of side effects.
- *Letronex*, a drug to treat irritable bowel syndrome in women, was withdrawn by the manufacturer *Smith Kline* in 2000, because of some fatal cases.
- HRT (*Hormone Replacement Therapy*) found to be dangerous for women who have coronary heart disease (CHD). Thromboembolism[295] and gallbladder disease can follow.[296]
- High doses of *Vioxx*, which we mentioned already, triples risks of heart attacks and sudden cardiac death.[297]
- In the year 2004, eighty thousand people went to emergency rooms with prescription drug overdoses (usually tranquilizers, like *Valium* and sedatives).

294 Michelle Meadows, "Why Drugs get pulled off the Market," http://www.fda.gov/fdac/features/2002/102_drug.html

295 Thromboembolism: the blocking of a blood vessel by a blood clot dislodged from its site of origin

296 http://www.healthcentral.com/ency/408/guides/000010.html

297 "FDA accused of silencing Vioxx warnings," see http://www.msnbc.msn.com/id/6205699

- Some long-term studies proved that drugs against "bad" cholesterol produce "cancer" in most animals, "and they may do it in human beings also."[298] Thirteen cases of breast cancer were reported in a test group taking the drug *Mecavor*, just one year after treatment caused death in another test group.

Dr. Uffe Ravskov concludes: "In human beings, the effects of cancer-producing chemicals are not seen before the passage of decades."… "Taking all experiments together, mortality from heart disease after treatment with these drugs was unchanged and the total mortality increased."[299]

- The drug *Warfarin*, a blood thinning agent, can be dangerous if taken at the same time as *aspirin*. The drug can lead to fatal bleeding in elderly people.[300]
- A high blood pressure drug combined with *Valium* can cause mental problems.
- Arthritis drugs often react with coffee or alcohol and can damage the stomach.
- *Diuretics* combined with heart medication can be dangerous.
- Eye *drops* for glaucoma can interact with diabetes and asthma drugs.[301]
- And what is it with our "famous aspirin"?

298 Uffe Ravnskov, "New cholesterol guidelines for converting healthy people into patients" http://www.ravnskov.nu/ncep_guidelines

299 Uffe Ravnskov, ibid. p. 4

300 http://www.bmj.com/cgi/content/full/325/7368/828

301 Idem.

In fact, one can read a totally different "success-story" of this medication. Here are the facts: "A reported 40,000 people die each year from the use of over-the-counter painkillers like aspirin."[302]

Author and nutritionist Mike Adams talks about "brainwashing" and the propaganda of the pharmaceutical industry when it comes to aspirin. But he is not the only voice. Reuters (Health) warned: "Stomach ulcers can arise from long-term use of aspirin."[303] Mike Adams puts it clearer, "Popping 14 or more aspirin tablets a week results in an 86% increase in the risk of contracting pancreatic cancer."[304]

Adams points to the "obscenely large profits, year after year" which are generated with aspirin and continues; "aspirin is also blamed for tens of thousands of death each year due to gastrointestinal bleeding." In the January 7 issue 2004 of the *Journal of the National Cancer Institute*, one also could read warnings against regular use of aspirin and the associated increased risk of pancreatic cancer. Women taking aspirin more than 20 years have a 58% increased risk of pancreatic cancer.[305]

So let us repeat:

- Many drugs do have side effects.
- Drugs are not tested long enough resulting in side effects coming to light only after many years.
- A high dose of a drug can kill.
- A wrong drug can kill.
- Drugs can have dangerous interactions, and one drug can suddenly react with another drug and cause disease – even death.

302 Mike Adams, "Aspirin and painkiller drugs cause widespread stomach ulcer," http://www.newstarget.com/000202.html

303 http://uk.reuters.com/article/governmentfilingsnews/idUKN1928836020061219

304 Mike Adams, "Long term aspirin use leads to pancreatic cancer," Sept. 15, 2004, http://www.naturalnews.com/000688.html

305 Source: http://sciencedaily.com/releases/2004/01/040107074621.htm

ADR

There is malpractice by doctors, hospitals, nurses, and pharmacy when it comes to drugs, without a doubt. Yes, an entirely desperate effort is going on so that reports about ADR (adverse drug reactions) are done more carefully. But consider this: a doctor who accidentally kills a patient with a drug will not always be very happy to report this, because HE is the one who administrated the drug. So the report system is inefficient, not to say that the interpretation of reports is often influenced by people who have a vested interest in a drug remaining on the market as long as possible.

In addition, adverse drug reactions are not even defined everywhere in the same way. The FDA states: "***Adverse events*** are defined by the FDA as *any unfavorable and unintended diagnosis, symptom, sign (including an abnormal laboratory finding), syndrome or disease which either occurs during the study, having been absent at baseline, or, if present at baseline, appears to worsen.*"[306]

The WHO defines it differently: "unexpected harm arising from a justified action where the correct process was followed for the context in which the event occurred. Recurrence of a known adverse reaction may be preventable (such as an allergic reaction to a drug, by avoiding re-exposure). A **side effect** is a known effect, other than that primarily intended, relating to the pharmacological properties of a medication. An example of an adverse reaction would be unexpectedly getting neutropenia (an abnormal decrease in the infection-fighting white blood cells in the blood commonly caused as a side effect by chemotherapy treatment) when that particular drug is not known to have this effect. An example would be when nausea, pruritus (severe itching of the skin) or urinary retention are encountered as side effects when morphine has been given to alleviate pain."[307]

But in spite of the different definitions, here is the situation: we face a huge under-reporting when it comes to drug reactions

306 http://www.nihtraining.com/ohsrsite/irb/attachments/5-10_serious_adverse_event_rep.htm

307 http://www.who.int/patientsafety/taxonomy/Report_Delphi_Survey_ICPS.pdf

because doctors fail to fill in these ADR forms due to complacency, ignorance, and perhaps guilt that their prescribed treatment has caused harm.

Also stated by the same source: "Only 5 to 10% of actual cases are believed to be reported," because, when multiple drugs are taken, who would know which one caused the side effects? Some ADR have a silent nature or a long-term nature. Damage to the kidney or the liver can happen over a long period of time. In other words, we are only looking at the tip of the iceberg. One doesn't need to be a prophet to foresee a great deal of medication scandal coming up in the future, and plenty of court cases.

But what is Big Pharma's concern about all that? Well, Big Pharma has its lawyers, a host of lawyers, which take care of these problems. Big Pharma is much more concerned when it comes to a point that a brand name, a drug protected by law, cannot be used exclusively anymore, and when the competition can move into the same market. Then Big Pharma goes wild. All sorts of strategies suddenly take place to do everything within their rights to protect a market and billions of dollars. Then Big Pharma loses patent protection and branded sales drop as much as 80%. Panic! So "creative strategies" are invented; the blockbuster drug has to be protected by all means. Sometimes, the pharmaceutical companies enter into manufacturing and distribution gentlemen-agreements with a generic drug company before a patent is about to expire.[308] Ohhhh – bestseller-pills have to be protected by all means! With "flanking strategies" and with defense strategies, litigation is used, turning patients quickly to a "next generation drug" – a practice know as "evergreen." Deals, which will never see the light, take place behind the backs of the public. Top Brand Names – that is everything.

---

308 http://drugtopics.modernmedicine.com/drugtopics/content/printContentPopup.jsp?id=121720

RANKING

There is an exact ranking of brand names, of which the pharmaceutical industry is very proud. Just read the first 33 names in the table below; these drugs made over 1 billion dollars in the year 2006.[309]

2006 Rank	Product	Total dollars (add 000)
1	Lipitor	$6,577,810
2	Nexium	4,060,286
3	Prevacid	3,305,778
4	Advair Diskus	3,105,780
5	Singulair	2,460,929
6	Effexor XR	2,246,965
7	Plavix	2,231,825
8	Zocor	2,171,312
9	Norvasc	2,149,017
10	Lexapro	2,098,794
11	Seroquel	2,074,734
12	Protonix	2,020,865
13	Ambien	1,938,649
14	Actos	1,926,293
15	Zoloft	1,772,599
16	Wellbutrin XL	1,670,516
17	Avandia	1,664,459
18	Risperdal	1,656,891
19	Zyprexa	1,536,167
20	Topamax	1,520,472
21	Toprol XL	1,471,881
22	Vytorin	1,469,209
23	Fosamax	1,427,165
24	Abilify	1,417,106
25	Levaquin	1,409,195
26	Lamictal	1,326,844
27	Celebrex	1,326,177
28	Lotrel	1,292,863
29	Zyrtec	1,163,312
30	Coreg	1,158,322
31	Valtrex	1,150,247
32	Zetia	1,139,638
33	Adderall XR	1,131,834

309 http://www.drugtopics.com/drugtopics/data/articlestandard//drugtopics/072007/405100/article.pdf

SOCIAL SIDE EFFECTS

The effects of drugs on the society at large are another factor. It has long since been known that alcohol and drug abuse costs the USA billions of dollars every year. Criminal behaviors, violence, job loss, financial destitution, all of these are the side effects of drugs. We have premature death, impaired productivity, motor vehicle crashes and repeatedly more crimes. Who pays this bill? We do! We have increasingly more "iatrogenic" diseases. My God, why don't we just say that doctors kill, and cause disease instead of saying "iatrogenic" disease?

Nevertheless, sleeping pills are an attractive market. And who wants to give up on the billions of dollars that is profited with aspirin, Viagra, and all the other blockbuster-drugs we spoke of: drugs for the young, drugs for the old, drugs for athletes, drugs for the whole population? Certainly, not the pharmaceutical industry.

So what is the real scandal here?

The real scandal is that hardly anyone knows the *actual* order of magnitude of our drug-society: we even take drugs with our food whether we want to or not. Most food industries work with chemical substances that sometimes have the same effect as a *drug*. When we eat meat today, we eat a lot of antibiotics and hormones at the same time. Poultry, pigs, calves, cattle – they are to a large degree fed with drugs and hormones; poultry averages more so than cattle, by the way.

In other words, there are side effects from sources never envisioned. One could call it side effects of side effects. Now hardly anyone knows the true proportion of those side effects of side effects. Why? Because it is not known, in the first place, that we are drugging ourselves continuously with "normal" food and "normal" beverages.

Another example: caffeine....

COFFEE

"Wake up and smell the coffee" takes on a new meaning when one has a look at just what caffeine does to the body. As well as many other harmful chemicals, coffee contains caffeine, a stimulant to the nervous system, and is considered a drug and rightly so. In fact, it is a psychoactive drug, which means it affects the mind, mood and behavior.[310] Consider how many times a person reaches for a cup of coffee when they are feeling down and needs a "pick-me-up." And then how many people are there that just can't get started in the morning without their cup of coffee or two? It seems, then, that caffeine gives a person energy, an emotional lift, and sharpens the mind. But let's explore this further and see if this is true.

First what is caffeine? Many substances contain this drug: coffee, tea, chocolate, and cocoa. In fact, caffeine is found in more than 80 species of plants.[311] Incredible! Caffeine is even added to many of our foods and medicines today. Look at the ingredients on many soda cans and chocolate bars. There we will find caffeine. Even certain yogurts and frozen desserts have caffeine. Medicines have caffeine added to them as is seen in this list:

- Cold and cough medications have caffeine combined with ASA and/or codeine
- Migraine and other headache treatment medicines (*Fiorinal, Fioricet*)
- Pain relievers such as *Anacin, Vanquish, Excedrin, Midol, Darvon, Synalgas-DC*, and *DGA*
- Muscle relaxants (*Norgesic, Forte*)
- Cold/allergy treatments (*Coryban-D*)
- Diuretics (*Aqua-ban*)
- Pep pills (*No Doz, Vivarin*)

---

310 Stephen Cherniske, M.S., *Caffeine Blues,* (New York: Warner Books, 1998), p. 46

311 Stephen states in his book "caffeine is a biological poison used by plants as a pesticide." Eating the plant will cause damage to the central nervous system of the predator and can prove lethal. *Caffeine Blues,* (New York: Warner Books, 1998), pp. 16 – 17.

It might not be a surprise then to know that caffeine is the most widely used drug in the world by both children and adults. Americans, themselves, consume over 420 million cups of coffee in one day making them the largest coffee consumers in the world.[312] In fact 90% of American adults drink caffeinated beverages. That's a large percentage that uses this drug.

And this brings us to these questions: is this drug harmless? Are there side effects? Does it really lift a person's mood, sharpen the mind or give an energy boost? And also, importantly, is it addictive?

There are definitely side effects as pointed out in the book *Caffeine Blues* and on the website *Facts about Drugs – Caffeine.* Caffeine raises blood pressure by stimulating the heart and yet constricting the blood vessels leading to the heart and increases the chemical homocysteine[313] willy-nilly that damages the artery walls.

With caffeine there is an ulcer risk as it irritates the stomach linking. It even causes a certain type of cancer and adrenal exhaustion, and creates hormone imbalances. The liver does not find it easy to reduce this toxin as it is rapidly absorbed by every organ and tissue in the body. So it is fast-acting and lasts for some time. In fact, it takes 15 minutes for the caffeine to act in the body, 12 hours to detoxify one cup of coffee and seven days to decaffeinate the blood of habitual coffee drinker.[314] Especially in combination with some drugs, normal antibiotics for example, the detoxification of caffeine is inhibited. "Researchers warn that ingestion of caffeine while taking such drugs can increase risk for liver disease, cardiac arrhythmias, and even epilepsy."[315]

312 Ibid. p. 15

313 Homocysteine is an amino acid used normally by the body in cellular metabolism and the manufacture of proteins. Elevated concentrations in the blood are thought to increase the risk for heart disease by damaging the lining of blood vessels and enhancing blood clotting.

314 Ibid. p.20 R.N. Warren, "Metabolism of Xanthenes Alkaloids in Man," *Journal of Chronalography*, 1969; 40, pp.468 – 69

315 Stephen Cherniske, *Caffeine Blues*, (New York: Warner Books, 1998), p. 54

As well, coffee today reduces the brain's ability to solve problems, increases the risk of gastrointestinal disease, increases the chance of having a heart attack or stroke, suppresses the immunity and causes one to age faster. This is especially true since we are living in a chemical and poisoned environment, and since we are usually over-medicated. It must be mentioned here, however, that recently newer findings have suggested that caffeine may be beneficial for the heart. This will be proven out over time.

What about the argument, then, that caffeine gives energy? How does it do that? And is it worth the side effects to have that energy? Good questions. Most coffee drinkers have that cup of coffee for the perceived energy it gives. And it works. At least for a while. But caffeine is the major cause of fatigue and it also interferes with the normal sleep pattern. The drug creates energy by creating tension. Tension results in fatigue and in the long run the result will be less energy, not more. How about that for a stab in the back? Gradually, more and more coffee will be needed to produce this energy and at the same time the adrenal glands become exhausted and function non-optimally. Adrenal exhaustion brings on profound tiredness. Thus the energy derived from caffeine is a façade. Another knife in the back.

How about mood enhancer? A person does feel much happier after a cup of coffee, wouldn't you say? Again, we are looking at a short-term effect and a long-term curse. After steady consuming of coffee, the final effect is a let down. Caffeine is linked to depression, anxiety and even to panic attacks.[316]

That leaves us with the argument that it sharpens the mind. Again we see that caffeine only increases sensory activity so that it appears the mind is more alert. In actual fact, caffeine decreases the overall mental activity. Studies showed that college students who were given 100 milligrams of caffeine did not do as well on tests compared to students who were given a placebo.[317]

316 Ibid. pp. 97 – 98

317 Ibid. p. 120

So with all these side effects there is yet one more question regarding coffee. Is it addictive? Well, here we see that someone who wants to stop drinking coffee suffers withdrawal symptoms as with any other addictive drug. They suffer headaches, depression, anxiety and fatigue, to name a few. The answer to this is yes.

Now imagine what amount of scientific research would be necessary to research just the interaction of *caffeine* with other drugs.

And this is just one single drug. We haven't talked about alcohol (here some interactions with medical drugs are known, but are all interactions known?). We didn't speak about tobacco; we didn't cover modern designer drugs or street drugs. We didn't mention the interaction between one medical drug and another medical drug extensively, because who can really know ALL those interactions.

How about when we take three drugs – two don't interact, but the third one does, and only when those two drugs are taken together? What about when we take 5 or 6 drugs and drink a cup of coffee? When we are at five, six, or seven drugs, the theoretical mathematical possibilities are astronomical. In theory, chemical scientific research could suddenly and literally find hundreds of dangers.

There will be, in fact, a new science one day, called SIDE EFFECTS. Already today, we have side effects of side effects. But soon we will have side effects of side effects of side effects.

Can anyone *imagine* the interaction of medication – drugs with food-drugs? Again: many Americans have to be hospitalized *because* of drugs. In hospitals, more drugs are given, and more mistakes are done, at least in many cases. The allegedly "ethical" drug companies produce these drugs – these medications. So we are surrounded by drugs, in food, in prescription drugs, and in over-the counter-drugs; we are surrounded by side effects and side effects of side effects.

SIDE EFFECTS OF SIDE EFFECTS

Did you know that there already exists a whole *science* on how to avoid dangerous drug interactions? In other words, know-how had to be developed just because drugs can react badly on another drug![318] But what, may one ask, happens when six drugs are taken simultaneously? This is often the case today with the old and the elderly. But even other people may make this mistake.

Alcohol for example is so *normal* today, that just taking one additional drug alone can have lethal consequences.

But the situation is even worse. Some drugs can have horrible side effects when taken together with certain food and, yes, hold your hat, even together with vitamins. There is currently a complete science developed on which food one should eat when one is on a particular drug.

Who is able to know all this? And again: just look at the mathematical side. Who has ever established the exact long-term consequences of taking six drugs simultaneously? Add different types of food and beverages, which may be deadly or result in horrible side effects, and we have over 100 possible situations. Do you think the pharmaceutical industry will test those 100 plus combinations in a long-term trial? Ha, Ha! One can only laugh cynically. Impossible!

The situation gets unbelievably complicated. And since more and more drugs are developed, nobody (repeat nobody) can control this situation anymore. We enter into an era of wild, crazy, chemical (read pharmaceutical) overload in which there is the side of effects of side effects, as one may call it, in an untested area. And often no one is aware of that. Can the single human being, not being an expert, have control over those side effects of side effects? Impossible! Even experts can do that only to a degree, because the mathematical combinations are too high.

If one buys over-the-counter remedies for a simple cold there may be substances that can be hazardous when taken together with

---

318 Joe Graedon and Teresa Graedon, *Dangerous Drug Interactions*, (New York: St. Martins Paperbacks, 1999)

certain antidepressants. *Prozac* can interact with antidepressants like: *Desyrel, Trofranil, Norpramin, Pamelor. Prozac* can interact with pain relievers, like *Talwin*, with *anti-anxiety agents* like *Valium* and *Xanax*, and with major tranquilizers like *Haldol.*[319]

It can be lethal. Case histories do exist. But even the healthiest food, like broccoli and spinach, superstar vegetables so to say, can be dangerous when a person takes a blood-thinning drug like Coumadin (Graedon, pg 64). Suddenly milk can be harmful; coffee of course, but also pudding.

If someone takes acne medicine (like *Accutane*) and vitamin A at the same time, this can increase toxicity in his body. Antibiotics can mess up with vitamin K. If he takes blood pressure medicines (like *Accupril, Altace, Capoten*, etc.) taking potassium at the same time can give him too much potassium and can be dangerous.

Asthma drugs interfere with Alzheimer's disease drugs. We could go on for a few hours. For the side effects of side effects of *Viagra* we can do a whole study of chemistry at the university. Read Joe Graedon's book and it will give a bit of an idea what we are up against today. To say it is wild is an understatement; it is lethal.

But all that we hear from the pharmaceutical industry (as a justification) is that it is so expensive to develop drugs, new drugs. Ha, even this is a lie.

"The industry's best-kept secret is that it's not very innovative at all. In 2002 the Food and Drug Administration approved 78 new drugs, of which only seven were truly innovative."[320]

Well, this may be *one* big secret, but certainly the *bigger* secret is the fact that this overload of drugs ruins our society completely. The FDA usually keeps some reports of Adverse Drug Events and Adverse Drug Reactions confidential for a time before acting.

---

319 Ibid. p. 25

320 Marcia Angell, physician and former editor of the New England, *Journal of Medicine*, now a senior lecturer in social medicine at Harvard University Medical School. See her book *The Truth about the Drug Companies: How They Deceive Us and What to Do about it*, (Random House) and see AARP Bulletin, Sept 2004, p. 18.

Despite the fact that there are some minor efforts to improve the reports of ADR, we are *not* hitting the real point. The real point (let us repeat the true scandal) is the side effects on our society, the *whole* society. So the actual scandal is *not* that drugs are too expensive. The actual scandal is *not* that one cannot buy drugs cheaply in Canada or that billions of dollars are earned by the pharmaceutical industry. The actual scandal is *not* that new drugs seldom get developed. The *actual* scandal is the fact that we get drugged, systematically, bit by bit. The whole culture moves in the direction of a drug society. We create drug personalities, and tomorrow we end up with a new type of Homo sapiens. We are facing a planet that is poisoning and drugging itself with chemicals and drugs, drugs, drugs. A new *type of man* is the actual scandal, a *dying race*.

So what is the solution?

THE SOLUTION

Well, the solution is certainly not to establish some more controls of the pharmaceutical industry. The FDA (the Food and Drug Administration, located in Rockville, Maryland) is obviously not doing the job.

The German newspaper Der Spiegel stated that, with the Vioxx scandal, the reputation of the FDA is gone. And he asks the question: are the managers of the FDA working too closely together with the pharmaceutical industry? The tests are too short; sometimes a new medication is put on the market after only a few months.

Vioxx again? Well what has happened with our highly acclaimed *Vioxx* medication? During the research for this book, the number of cases that reported horrible side effects from this medication continued to rise. In Germany alone, 7,000 patients claimed to have experienced side effects such as stroke and heart attack. In the USA, 14,000 people went public and took their cases to court. Cases of mortality were also reported. The USA American pharmaceutical firm, *Merck,* did not have a good time at all.

Merck had earned 2.5 billion dollars from the sales of the blockbuster *Vioxx* in 2003 alone. But the increased heart risks have now been repeatedly documented. In one single day, the value of Merck on the stock exchange sank 5.2 billion dollars, after a judge in Texas ruled that the relatives of a deceased *Vioxx* patient be awarded $253 million settlement. (Der Spiegel, 41/2006, pg. 94)

The Spiegel reported about missing time in the FDA and fear of juniors in relation to the seniors.[321] And Big Pharma itself, of course, is utterly unable to publish neutral, objective, or scientific findings, because billions are at stake for them.

So it would be completely wrong to strengthen the FDA, to fire the head of the FDA and replace with another, or give Big Pharma the responsibility for the surveillance of their products. The worse solution would be to spend more money in a direction that has utterly failed.

A real solution would be to write a hundred more books about the sins of the pharmaceutical industry and the FDA, bring *everything* to light. A real solution would be to hold Big Pharma accountable for the unbelievable damage that has been done so far.

A real solution would be to investigate the lives and "scientific findings" of those doctors, professors and researchers who are directly responsible for killing people in the end or for making them even sicker. A real solution would be for many more lawyers engaging in an ethical fight against Big Pharma and taking down those giants.

A real solution would be to investigate the money that is spent for some politician and remove every politician who is directly or indirectly corrupted by the money of the pharmaceutical industry. Politicians have to represent the people, not Big Pharma.

A real solution would mean making it unbelievably hard to launch any new pharmaceutical product. It would have to be checked for side effects for at least 10 years by three neutral institutions, which have no connections whatsoever to Big Pharma – their location and personnel unknown. And when anyone from

321 Der Spiegel, 6/2005

these institutions meets privately with one of those pharmaceutical affiliates, he would lose his job on the spot. A person who once worked for Big Pharma is unqualified of course.

The real solution would be to give true information to the public and tell them the truth that drugs seldom help and should be avoided by any means as long as possible. Pushing alternative healing methods must be the talk of the day.

The real solutions would also be to check the efficiency of those alternative healing methods by objective and neutral field studies.

The real solution would mean taking the pharmaceutical industry down to the size of about 3% of what it is now. The real solution embraces to cut all this fraud and corruption, and utterly change the direction mankind currently walks regarding *health.* The real solution would be to educate doctors in such thorough, nutritional therapies, so that diseases are stopped before they can begin. The real solution would embrace an utter reform of the medicinal studies in universities.

A real solution would endeavor to turn this world toward a completely different direction, away from drugs and obsessive operations, away from this gigantic health industry. It would eradicate suppressive, nutritional food companies and forbid chemical, water, and air pollution.

A real solution would mean an utterly new way of living and a much higher standard of life.

Let's take a look at that.

10. FIGHTING DRUGS AND FINDING ALTERNATIVES (1): HEALTHY NUTRITION

It would not be fair to talk about the horrible side effects of drugs, without at least mentioning the alternatives to drugs. The know-how, in essence, of how to help oneself with the natural approach embraces a whole library. The common denominators are always the same: organic food, good water, exercise, and fresh air. But there are, in addition, lots and lots of wonder foods and nutritional supplements that work astonishingly well, in addition to vitamins, enzymes and minerals. Entire books exist to tell us how to fight arthritis, asthma, cancer, constipation, depression, colds and flu's naturally, all the way down though the alphabet of diseases. Prostate disorders, menopause, osteoporosis, fatigue, overweight, rheumatism, heart disease, high blood pressure, answers to ulcers, diabetes and even hair loss and insomnia, can be treated naturally or prevented more optimally by natural approaches which are by average far less dangerous.[322] There is a host of know-how, from herbs and natural supplements[323] up to entire books talking about good fats that can heal and bad fats that can kill.[324] Good fats increase cardiovascular health and immune function.

Enormous books are on the market that just tell us how to create a safe home by avoiding everyday toxins and harmful household products, which are sometimes covertly responsible for a disease.[325]

There even exists in one work an unbelievable amount of know-how of how to avoid disease and if one is sick, how to turn

---

322 For example, Joseph J. Sweere, *Golden Rules for Vibrant Health in Body, Mind, and Spirit*, (North Bergen, NJ: Basic Health Publications, 2004) or *Amazing Medicines, the Drug Companies Don't Want You to Discover*, (Tempe, Arizona: University Medical Research publishers, 1993).

323 Linda Skidmore-Roth, *Mosby's Handbook of Herbs and Natural Supplements*, (St. Louis, Missouri: Mosby Inc, 2001)

324 Udo Erasmus, *Fats that Heal, Fats that Kill*, (Burnaby, BC, Canada: Alive Books, 1993)

325 DebraLynn Dadd, *Home Safe Home*, (New York: Penguin Putman, 1997)

back the wheel of time to regain health naturally. In fact, so much good news exists that one could fill a hundred books with it and one would not be finished.

DRUGS VERSUS ALTERNATIVE HEALING

Look around and you will see that there is a complete movement operating against drugs. Everywhere you look you will find good news, whether it has to do with the topic of heart disease, eye problems, autoimmune diseases, osteoporosis, lung diseases, diabetes, or chronic fatigue.[326] Nutritional healing is the talk of the day, and we are probably just at the beginning of a new age of medicine, if we choose to take this route. Medical heretics, like Dr. Robert S. Mendelsohn,[327] tell us again and again what horrible side effects drugs have, and that there are a lot of alternative medicines that are not dangerous and are without side effects.

Dr. Mendelsohn, a doctor who once worked as an M.D., states, "I believe that more than 90% of modern medicine could disappear from the face of the earth – doctors, hospitals, drugs, and equipment, and the effect on our health would be immediate and beneficial." (pg. XI)

He talks at length about the danger of drugs. "Medicine is neither an art nor a science. It's a religion." (pg. xiii) He guesses that 90% of the surgery done is a waste of time in energy, money and life – and he is an insider! He knows that doctors work covertly or openly for drug companies, making a good buck and telling the public what the drug companies want them to say. He knows about all those faked "scientific findings." No word is greater than the word *science*. Who pays the most may use it. And he gives (after a long life of being a medical doctor) the advice to look for alternatives.

---

326 See Ray D. Strand, M.D., *What Your Doctor Doesn't Know About May be Killing You*, (Nashville, TN: Thomas Nelsen Publishers, 2002)

327 Robert S. Mendelsohn, *Confessions of a Medical Heretic*, (Chicago, Illinois: Contemporary Books, 1979)

There exists alternative medicine in such a large order of magnitude, one cannot even imagine, because there is so much know-how in existence. Just plant-based medicines, thousands of years old, give literally thousands of new possible substances that can help.[328]

Right now, while reading this book, new plant-based medications are detected, because the healing properties of some Amazon plants or far-eastern plants or Inner African plants never before detected, now find their way into our "knowledge book" of the West. Every year a new break-through is made in the area of plant-based medicine.

Yes, one can reverse the drug cycle. One can undo the horrifying effects of drugs. One can live without drugs. The most exciting message of this book is that perhaps techniques exist, which are more powerful than the most powerful drug. When it comes to health, there are, in fact, literally hundreds of techniques in existence today that work like a bomb. Silently, without the noisy advertisement of the school of medicine, geniuses developed healing techniques that were not in existence 100 or 200 years ago.

Of course, it is not this book's purpose to talk about each and every technique; we have to concentrate on the subject of *drugs*. But we can talk about some breathtaking techniques that can make a sick body healthy again; which can make a drugged body a drug-free body again.

The first step consists of a change in diet because there are plenty of drugs and chemicals in our daily nutrition, as we mentioned earlier. So let's take that subject up before we talk about some amazing drug detoxification programs.

NUTRITION

The authors guess that of the so-called schools of medicine only 0.1% is valuable. Yes, we need this medicine in case of an emergency,

328 C.W. Fetrow, Juan R. Avila, *Complementary and Alternative Medicines*, (Philadelphia: Lippencott Williams and Wilkins), reedited and brought up to date regularly

but in general, those schools of medicines are neglecting the basics. What are the basics? Simply – nutrition. Nutrition techniques are 100% applicable to *every* person.

Nutrition is so sophisticated today, so highly developed and so intelligent as never before. The only problem one encounters is the fact that there are 1001 nutrition-gurus. Every year a new guru arises like a phoenix from the ashes, and says he has found the ultimate truth. Thus, statements about nutrition are contradictory. Why? Because billion-dollar industries earn a vast amount of money here. Like doctors who can be bribed, nutritionists can be *persuaded* to tell the public that, for example, sugar gives one energy and is good for one. In fact, there are confusion-techniques in existence that one should know about. These techniques are worthwhile to examine; the observation is very revealing. Let us take the famous sugar example. Actually everybody knows today that sugar isn't good for his or her health, right? So how is sugar sold? And which CONFUSION-TECHNIQUES are used?

CONFUSION TECHNIQUE NO. 1: THE SCIENTIFIC TOUCH

A sure way to confuse someone is to pelt him with scientific words that are not part of the daily vocabulary. Being unsure of the meaning of these scientific terms, he feels a little stupid. This tactic is very mean and very tricky. And it works. One way to hide the fact that sugar for example is present in a lot of food is to call it by a different name, *carbohydrate*. Of course, sugar is *also* a carbohydrate. The carbohydrates embrace all forms of sugar, but carbohydrates include other food too. But by saying *carbohydrates*, one is lured into a false feeling of not eating sugar. The computation goes: "*I'm not eating sugar. I'm eating carbohydrates*." This is called positioning. It allows sugar to hitch a free ride on the coat tails of other carbohydrates such as legumes, barley, wheat, pasta, rice and vegetables. Again, sugar is also a carbohydrate. Lots of foods are carbohydrates. But by saying that it is a carbohydrate, one has avoided using the "S" word. Do you see the trick for what it is?

One can also give the chemical formula for it, another surefire way to make sure that no one will understand it. This fools lots of people. Here is a little poem to reinforce the concept.

Little Willie was a chemist.
Little Willie is no more.
What he thought was H_2O,
Was really H_2SO_4

If someone hasn't studied chemistry, it is easy to be misled and misinformed about this. While H_2O is water, H_2SO_4 is sulfuric acid, and it can melt the skin. There are other subterfuges. Milk sugar can be called "lactose." "Maltose" is malt sugar. "Dextrose" is synthetically derived from starch, and is also called corn sugar. Using scientific nomenclature can hide the fact that it is sugar, but the fact is that all of it is refined sugar, derived from sugar cane, sugar beets or other sugar sources.

CONFUSION TECHNIQUE NO. 2: THE NAME GAME

Basically, the whole thing is very, very simple. All words ending with the letters "-ose" have to do with sugar. Here are some examples.

Dextrose is corn sugar.
Fructose is fruit sugar.
Lactose is milk sugar.
Maltose is malt sugar.
Maple sugar is fructose.
Sugar is sugar. Sugar, sugar, sugar!

Well, what about *glucose*? Yes, we do need *glucose* for life. But the body makes the glucose all by itself. It does not need assistance from the Imperial Sugar or American Crystal Sugar Company or the Fidel Castro Sugar Company. The body makes glucose out of the meat, grains, vegetables and whole fruits that one eats naturally.

It simply does not need all of those "-oses." The whole idea of this "name game" is to convey to each one of us the idea that the speaker or writer knows more about this stuff than we do; that we should not think for ourselves; and we should buy more sug – oops – we mean carbohydrates with high fructose corn syrup. It is designed to keep us from thinking for ourselves. It is designed to stop us from handling our sugar addiction.

CONFUSION TECHNIQUE NO. 3: POSITIVE ASSOCIATION VALUE

Positive Association Value is an advertising term. It has nothing to do with what is good or bad. It is just the use of words to better *position* the product that is being sold. Whether it is smoking cigarettes ("Hey kids, look at how cool Joe Camel is"), or joining the Army ("I am an army of one – you can see my strength"), it is the concept of positioning the product. Ethics and morals have nothing to do with it. We are all susceptible to this manipulation because of the daily barrage of advertising that tells us that something is okay. This is done with salvos of advertising slogans and scripts designed to better position the product, using powerful imagery, and to counter any efforts at reasonable education.

The technique is fascinating. One overworked word is *natural*. If one wants to sell something, it is labeled with the word *natural*. But wait a minute. This word doesn't mean anything. Everything is *natural*. Even heroin is natural. Cocaine is natural. Even artificial substances can be linguistically perverted into being "natural." After all, many chemicals are found in nature. We just take these natural chemicals, mix them together, heat them to 2,000 degrees centigrade, under enormous pressure, remove an electron or two, and then combine it with thirteen similarly altered natural chemicals and see – pass the gas mask please – it's all perfectly "natural."

The same is true of the word *biological*. A bio-product. Everything is animal, vegetable or mineral. So everything is *biological*, in a manner of speaking. The implication is that it's good for you. The reality is that even the deadly Ebola virus[329] and its various mutations are bio-products. Picture a dark wizard making a potion to do some evil deed. Eye of newt, wing of bat and dead toads are all biological. Like the black wizard, the chemical companies take all kinds of products, including little known living things from the jungles of South America, and turn them into a holistic nightmare. Better living through chemistry, indeed! The ad men use good-sounding, positive words to trick one into buying something with a clear conscience, but it undermines one's health. The next confusion technique is also a malodorous use of language for private profit at the expense of the health of the general population.

CONFUSION TECHNIQUE NO. 4: REDEFINING WORDS

One of the biggest scams in history relates to the redefinition of the word "democracy." No one can say that he is against democracy. Thus, the word has come to be used in even the most dictatorial countries. Former East Germany was known as the "DDR," the "*Deutsche Demokratische Republik.*" Well, the Deutsche part was true – Deutsche means German. But it was neither a democracy nor a republic. It was exactly the opposite – a dictatorship.

One should look at the true meanings of words. Words are patient. Words are like empty bottles, waiting to be filled with a new significance. The old label is left on the bottle. It just has a new significance depending on how it is crafted. The dark side of this is that public relations specialists redefine words. They change the labels on the bottles to suit the particular needs of their clients rather than let the language grow in its own natural way. The public relations specialists who do this are like gangsters, accomplices in the overall caper of robbing us of our health in order to fill the coffers of their drug pushing masters.

329 Ebola virus: an extremely contagious virus that causes an acute, highly fatal hemorrhagic fever. It is spread through contact with bodily fluids or secretions of infected persons and by airborne particles.

This deceptive technique is not constrained to the public relations firms. The food companies themselves have engaged in a long history of altering the food to make it fit the definition. For instance, when holistic physicians and nutritionists discovered and promoted the benefits of eating brown rice, the food processing companies jumped on the bandwagon by taking white rice and dying it brown. Sure, it was brown rice, but it was not the healthful fiber filled natural brown rice that was the subject of the discovery. Another company sent old discolored shrimp, which could not be legally sold in the United States, out of the country. While overseas, the shrimp was bleached white again, and then shipped back into the U. S. where it was fraudulently sold as fresh shrimp. We know of these frauds because the perpetrators are caught. This brings us to the next confusion technique, another method of cooking the words to make the lie seem true.

CONFUSION TECHNIQUE NO. 5: DOUBLE MEANINGS

Let us again take up the innocent term *sugar*. *Blood sugar* this time. Yes, we all need blood sugar. *Glucose*. Scientifically spoken, with a stiff upper lip and a scientifically arrogant little smile on the lips, "*We need blood sugar*." Perhaps a white lab coat, even if it is just worn by a professional actor – the best actor that money can buy. Now comes the scam, "*Therefore, we need to consume more sugar*." No! No! No! Sugar and blood sugar are two totally different things. They couldn't be further apart. In both terms we do encounter the word "sugar." That doesn't mean that these things are chemically or biologically the same. They are worlds apart. Blood sugar has to do with correctly changing food into fuel for the body to use. Sure, sugar will influence blood sugar, but the influence is a negative influence. The two terms couldn't be more different in meaning.

These are the five primary confusion techniques, all designed to make one's head spin. There are great looking models, beautiful women and handsome men, renowned athletes, all telling us how important it is for us to eat this or that.

BRINGING IN THE BASICS: WHAT MAKES BODIES FLOURISH AND PROSPER

Again, realize that no subject is as confused as the subject of nutrition. Virtually every "authority" has a different "expert" opinion. There are more prophets in this field than in the Old Testament. For example, many a doctor – and actress! – have found success in penning quick weight loss books. What they all have in common is that they all know the "true secrets" of how to properly nourish our bodies. Never does a year go by without the release of a new best-selling tome disclosing the latest, hottest findings about nutrition.

These "authorities," of whatever stripe, always use their successes to "prove" that their "system" is the perfect one. Their error is the extrapolation that their "proven method" includes everyone and invalidates all other systems. Their "studies," when they bother to conduct them at all, do not involve enough participants to offer any sound statistical data about the validity of the trials and experiments. Scientifically, a valid discovery is one that can be successfully repeated over and over again. In other words, a valid discovery in the field of nutrition would mean that a large number of people could apply that discovery to themselves and the vast majority of them would be successful in achieving the expected benefit or result of the research.

We have heard and read a great deal about the "scientific evidence" of these nutrition and health "authorities." And rather than becoming more and more informed and enlightened about how to best take care of ourselves nutritionally, we have become more and more confused. In the worst-case scenario, we apply totally unhealthy principles and our physical well-being has deteriorated because of it.

PROTEIN

Let's start by taking a look at what food is all about. It may come as a pleasant surprise to find that this subject can be easily understood. There are really just two issues to consider.

Food is sorted into two large groups. These two groups are called "macronutrients" and "micronutrients."

Macronutrients and micronutrients – it really is very simple. Macronutrients are divided into protein, fat and carbohydrates. Micronutrients are vitamins, minerals and trace elements. Let's look at the macronutrients first. Remember, they are protein, fat and carbohydrates. Protein, to make things simple, is found mainly in fish, meat and eggs, and, to some degree, in vegetables and legumes. Protein is the building-block source for the body. It has been well established by extensive experimentation that the body cannot survive without protein. If protein is absent or insufficient, the body will lack energy (its organs and cells cannot be repaired) and it becomes tired. It will become ill and eventually die.

One might say protein, containing the amino acids, is factor #1 for survival. To put it enthusiastically, protein is life! Protein is literally the stuff of which bodies are made – along with water, of course. Anyone who tells us that protein is not essential is ignoring hundreds of scientific studies, not to mention common sense and simple observation. There are valid studies that one can live without sugar, of course. But protein? No, in the absence of protein, the body's health will deteriorate just as surely as it will suffer if exposed to the radioactive fallout from a nuclear bomb.

Protein stems from the Greek word *protos,* which means first. It can be taken quite literally. It is the first thing that the body needs. Chemically speaking, protein is a class of complex substances, which is mainly derived from animal sources. There are plant proteins as well, but animal foods are the most concentrated source. Proteins from animal foods also contain many essential micronutrients, such as Vitamins B_1, B_2, B_6 and B_{12}. Meat proteins also contain plenty of zinc and iron. Some of these vitamins and minerals can also be found in plant proteins.[330] The fat contained in animal proteins is also an important nutrient.

There are many nutrients that are contained in meat that the human body cannot produce. People who eat only plant-based proteins and do not take nutritional supplements, mainly amino acids, to supply them with the nutrients they are missing by not eating meat will eventually develop debilitating and dangerous nutritional deficiencies.

Meat is not the enemy!

FIRST SURPRISE: Meat can be an important protein source. Eating meat is the right thing to do. It provides energy.

SECOND SURPRISE: Of all the meat available on the market, 99%is low quality meat. Don't eat that meat!

And that's the long and the short of it.

While much of the meat supply is contaminated and toxic and most of the animals that provide this meat are abominably treated, there *are* safe and healthy meat products on the market and there are commercial farmers who treat the animals under their care decently and humanely. This *organic* meat is grass-fed and antibiotic and hormone free.[331] No chemicals; no drugs, in other words. It is important to understand why we can and should resolve these non-optimum meat issues by buying and consuming high quality meats. People who avoid all meat products may be protein deficient. A vegan must be aware of this and take care to monitor protein intake. They may also be devoted to a *low fat* diet. This means that they may not be eating enough healthy *omega 3 fats*, which, in turn,

330 Nicolai Worm, *Daily Meat*, (Hamburg: Hamburg Press, 2002)

331 By "organic," we mean food and meat produced without antibiotics, hormones, chemical fertilizers and other such biotechnology. Such food must not be treated with sewage sludge or exposed to irradiation or mingled with genetically modified organisms.

means that they are not sufficiently able to produce hormones and this can cause a disastrous chain reaction. The integrity of the cellular membranes is compromised, leading to deterioration. The cell's *immune responses* are weakened.

CARBOHYDRATES

Carbohydrates are the second biggest in the family of macronutrients. They are compounds that are composed of carbon, hydrogen and oxygen and includes sugars and starches. In the language of the mom who does the family grocery shopping, this group of nutrients includes such foods as pizza, pasta, potatoes, breads, cakes, candies, starchy vegetables and sweet fruits. About 70% of the foods that are eaten today are carbohydrates.

Carbohydrates are important. All one has to know is that there are **good** carbohydrates and **bad** carbohydrates. Simple! Good carbohydrates: corn bread made 100% from cornmeal for example, and bad carbohydrates: white bread, for example. Good carbohydrates: green vegetables; bad carbohydrates: sugar.

You see? The word *carbohydrates* alone doesn't say anything. It doesn't say anything about the *quality* of the carbohydrate. The *quality* – that is the kicker!

Therefore, the only carbohydrates that we would advise a person to eat are good carbohydrates. This is not because they are carbohydrates, which they are, of course, but because they contain many vitamins, minerals, and other micronutrients that one will need in order to rebuild and maintain good health.

Green vegetables, or corn bread are very good for us, providing we haven't developed an allergy to them. It could be said that they are whole, complex carbohydrates. These *complex carbohydrates* contain vitamins, minerals and fiber, which are vital to one's good health. The sugary or starchy *refined carbohydrates* do not because they (unlike their wholesome, whole-grain predecessors – which are very hard to come by these days) lack vitamins, enzymes and fiber.

The refining process has stripped away all of these nutrients. [332] It's important to understand that *refined carbohydrates* are something totally different than *complex carbohydrates*.

The word *carbohydrate* is a dangerous word. Remember the Confusion Techniques? Well, the word *carbohydrate* has a double meaning. It can mean something good and something bad.

Let us repeat *good carbs* (green vegetables) do not contain as much sugar and contain lots of other balancing factors like minerals and fiber. But *bad carbs* are starches, like white bread, or mashed potatoes, which convert directly into sugar in the body. So, the starchier the food, the *bad-er* it is as a carbohydrate. Green lettuce = good. Rice cakes = bad. There are lots of degrees of good and bad in between. A good glycemic index table[333] will lay it all out perfectly.

Anyway, complex carbohydrates or *good* carbohydrates, such as green vegetables, are very useful. Eat all of the fresh green vegetables you can get your hands on – spinach, celery, cabbage, asparagus, you name it. And eat corn bread.

The second big secret weapon in nutrition when someone wants to fight drugs and chemicals is the green vegetable, particularly the bitter green vegetables and corn bread. Again, the point is to only select *organic* vegetables. Otherwise, a person will be exposed to pesticides and other toxins that will not help him. He is, in a way, still close to drugs.

FATS

As you may recall, fats are another member of a trio of major food groups, called "macronutrients," which also include proteins and carbohydrates.

What is fat? How can we tell one type of fat from another? What does a person with health concerns need to know about fats in relation to his or her diet?

---

332 Sally Fallon, *Nourishing Traditions*, (San Diego, CA: ProMotion Publishing, 1995), p 15

333 A glycemic index is found on the Internet at http://www.diabetesnet.com/diabetes_food_diet/glycemic_index.php

One could say that there are good fats and bad fats. Good fats are organic, natural and unrefined. Bad fats are non-organic, unnatural and refined, to state it very simply.

But do we need fat at all? Yes, fats are important and good for us because they are formed in the cells and are another source of energy. Our bodies need fats in order to function properly. They are the parts of foods that are the *oils* or the *greasy stuff*. As well as coming from animal sources such as eggs, chicken or beef, they are also derived from plant sources such as avocados, olives, nuts and seeds.

Fats have several major functions in the body. In a body that is not addicted to refined carbohydrates, fats are burned slowly for fuel, like a thick oak log in a fireplace, unlike refined carbohydrates, which the body burns quickly like paper or dry kindling. The fats we consume are recombined to create one very essential fat, cholesterol. Cholesterol is used by the body to make many types of hormones. (Women who have been on fat restricted diets for a long period of time develop severe hormone imbalances.) When people consume too little fat they are likely to become depressed. A diet that is insufficient in nutritious fats will ultimately result in a weakened immune response. This means that the cells have become vulnerable to attack by viruses, bacteria and other invaders. A person in this condition is at risk for chronic viral, bacterial or yeast infections.

Fats are metabolized by being broken down in the body and then burned for fuel. So, technically, fats are considered to be *potential energy*.

Animal fats, of course, occur along with animal protein. That is why there is often a connection between a low fat diet and an insufficient intake of protein. People who maintain a low fat and low protein diet for too long sustain damage to their tissues and organs because the cells lose the ability to repair themselves in the absence of an adequate supply of protein. The excessive heat that is generated by the rapid metabolism of starches and sugars – the only food/energy source that such dieters allow themselves – further damages the body. This is much like a fireplace that is damaged by an overly large fire or an uncontrolled flue fire.

We don't mean to put anyone through a crash course in body chemistry, so we'll wrap it up by saying briefly what one needs to know about fat in the diet. Good fat is good, very good. Bad fats are very bad. But don't run out and buy margarine to melt on your spinach, please. The best source of fat is organic cold-pressed flax oil, coconut oil and olive oil. The other source of fats that one should eat comes from organic meat.

APPLICATION

So far the facts. The good news is: one can successfully treat people in an astonishing number of cases by just teaching them to eat well again. Just eat healthy, avoid sugar by all means and avoid refined carbohydrates. Avoid alcohol and any sort of drug. One of the authors of this book treated over 8000 patients so far. Lots of people can be healed by change of nutritional diet alone.

But it gets even more exciting!

VITAMINS AND MINERALS

The world was stunned. In 1912, Dr. Erik Fink, a Norwegian biochemist, isolated the first vitamin. In the same year, an English biochemist, I.G. Hopkins, conducted research that pointed in the same direction. In 1913, McCollum and Davis, two researchers at the University of Wisconsin, discovered that a substance found in egg yolks – which they called *vitamin A* – could successfully treat people of certain diseases.[334] Just like a miracle, it could make people well.

Nutritionists jumped for joy. At long last, one of life's deepest secrets was revealed! Man's search for the basic building blocks of nutrition was yielding results. The reputation of *science* was elevated dramatically because of these discoveries. The newly

334 For a good explanation of vitamins see Judith A. DeCava, *The Real Truth About Vitamins and Antioxidants,* (Columbus, GA: Brentwood Christian Press, 1996).

coined word *vitamin* became a hot topic of conversation. Vitamin stems from the Latin word *vita*, which means *life.*

In the months and years that followed, more and more vitamins were discovered. In short order, McCollum and Davis discovered ***B***, followed in quick succession by ***D***, ***E***, and ***K***. And so it went, through the alphabet.

It was pretty amazing stuff. People were electrified. Vitamin A could successfully treat bad eyesight. B_1 could reduce infections. B_6 was great for muscle problems. B_{12}'s healing powers were noted in relation to red blood cells and the nervous system. Vitamin C seemed to be a *miracle treatment*, proving itself to be effective against colds, infections and a host of other maladies. Vitamin D seemed to be very helpful in building strong bones. The possibilities were endless. Nutrition entered a Golden Age.

It seemed that science had triumphed over this riddle we call the human body. Vitamins were manufactured and distributed all over the world. In Japan, the United States, Germany and many other European countries, vitamins became the thing to have for people who were interested in maintaining good health. Even the pharmaceutical giants got into the vitamin game. Vitamins were big business and they were heavily promoted as the solution to every physical complaint or illness.

It make come as a shock to hear the real low-down on vitamins. But first, let us concentrate on some more good news. Yes, vitamins are, up to the present, the alternative to successfully handling maladies. They can't do everything, but they can do a lot. Since much of our food is processed, refined and laced with chemicals and preservatives, and since most of us are suffering today from one or the other form of nutritional depletion, it is wise to take vitamins (and minerals) daily. When one is sick, vitamins are a must. Now, to list all the possible good effects of vitamins is impossible because, again, this book is about drugs. But permit us to say this: B_1 can improve memory, B_3 cuts back the possibility of heart attack *by almost 30%*,[335] and B5 helps with stress. B_6 helps to

335 *Amazing Medicines*, ibid. p. 325

improve mental functions in general and is a super immune-builder. B_{12} aids in absorbing and learning new data and is responsible for energy. B Complex can even help raise the IQ. Vitamin C has at least 50 positive effects and is an IQ increaser as well. It helps with nerves and helps with memory improvement (why take dangerous drugs). Mega doses of Vitamin C can help infertile men and also seems to play a role in anti-cancer therapies. Vitamin E guards the nerves and is effective against narrowing of the arteries. Vitamin D is crucial for the immune system and may play a role in cancer prevention as well. And so we could go on and on, but the truth is that other authors have researched the power of vitamins already very well, so why compete with them? To make a long story short, vitamins can do at least three things:

(1) Vitamins can impede one from getting sick, and so one wouldn't have to take drugs.
(2) Vitamins can help one in getting well, without drugs.
(3) Vitamins can balance out the horrible side effects of some drugs.

Vitamins are, in short, the natural fighters against disease. They are much cheaper than most drugs, seldom have any side effects, and cannot be patented. However, there is a big BUT. It is hard to believe, but even around the topic of *vitamins* there already exists a new form of criminality. It's not enough to pop a few synthetic vitamins in the morning to give one the necessary nutrition. So let's let the cat out of the bag.

THE TRUTH ABOUT VITAMINS

TRUTH #1: Yes, the body does need vitamins. In fact, in view of the poor quality of the food supply that is available in the marketplace today, the body desperately needs them.

TRUTH #2: Yes, in some specific cases, just giving a high concentration of a good quality vitamin can bring about a healthy recovery within a patient. But these cases are few and far between, nowadays.

TRUTH #3: There is an enormous difference between a natural, living vitamin and a synthetic one. Advertising suggests that there is no difference; however, the chemically synthesized vitamins often contain only a fraction of the nutritional value of a vitamin derived from a natural source. Further, the body frequently is unable to assimilate synthetic vitamins.

TRUTH #4: Some vitamins must be precisely balanced with other vitamins. Otherwise, the body is incapable of absorbing and using the vitamins. Worse yet, it is possible to overdose on certain vitamins. This, of course, produces a very undesirable toxic reaction in the body.

TRUTH #5: There are some sleazy criminal manufacturers out there turning out some low quality vitamins. On top of that, there are some additives and fillers in vitamin tablets and capsules that cause allergic reactions in some people.

Here's a classic case, and it concerns an unlikely suspect – good old reliable vitamin C. *Ascorbic acid* or even *ascorbate* is not really vitamin C. It is only the anti-oxidant outer shell of the vitamin C complex molecule that protects the really valuable stuff that is real vitamin C. Now here's the kicker. Guess what these ascorbic acids and ascorbates are sometimes made from? Hold on to your hat. Cornstarch! And what does cornstarch break down into as soon as it hits the body? *Sugar!*

Here's another example. We sometimes hear people being told to take things like balanced B complex with 50 or 100 mgs or micrograms of each B vitamin. The problem is that this so-called balance does not appear like this anywhere in nature. It is a total falsehood. It often boosts energy in the beginning but slowly causes problems as these synthetic, out-of-natural-balance formulas create even more deficiencies.

We are sorry to have to say this about vitamins: what one hears is not necessarily what one gets.

DIFFERENTIATION

So if one is going to work with vitamins, the most important point is to differentiate. One has to differentiate between various types of vitamins. Probably never before in history has so much money been spent on the advertising and the purchasing of any merchandise with so little knowledge of the product itself on the part of either the seller or the buyer. Billions are being spent annually and most of the purchasers, jobbers, wholesalers, retailers, or direct-to-the-consumer salesmen do not know the difference between a synthetic, a crystalline or a true natural vitamin. They know little of how they are made, their characteristics, their attributes, their sources, their advantages or disadvantages, and how to tell one from the other by reading the label.

As far as our literature is concerned, "natural" means vitamins as found in natural foods, non-tampered with (not segregated, separated or isolated) in any way that might change their molecules – their biological or biochemical combinations, or their action – which usually means that only fiber and moisture are removed. Natural food vitamins are never highly concentrated. Nature is interested in balance not potency. This means that to get higher than normal potency, natural vitamins must be consumed in greater quantity. *Synthetic* and *crystalline* vitamins lend themselves to high potency concentration in a few small pills. Naturals must be used in greater quantity than one would with food.

Natural vitamins build slowly but exceedingly well, as nature always does. *Synthetics* can give a quick spasmodic spurt that may not be lasting. Naturals are nontoxic in any consumable quantity. Some synthetics may be very toxic. *Synthetics* are not a genuine food. Finally, naturals are much more expensive because they are perishable and every precaution must be taken to preserve their life and integrity. Synthetics are mostly *dead*, inert, and cheaper, and they present much less expensive handling problems. As with any inert material, greater mass production creates cheaper bargain prices. All labels of truly natural food concentrates should indicate the exact food source from which a vitamin is obtained.

Now let us give more exact definitions:

> CRYSTALLINE – means it had a natural food as its original source but probably was treated with various high powered chemicals, solvents, heat, and distillations to reduce it down to one specific pure crystalline vitamin or amino-acid. It is no longer natural. It no longer has its synergists (enzymes, coenzymes, minerals, mineral activators, and co-vitamin helpers). It has been reduced to a pure simple crystalline powder.

> SYNTHETIC – means that in the laboratory, the scientist has attempted to reconstruct the exact structure of the crystalline molecule by *putting together* or chemically combining molecules from other known sources. Chemically, therefore, there is no difference between the synthetic and the crystalline. As a vitamin, there is no difference between the two. The crystalline may have a slight advantage in that it is difficult to reduce any natural product to an absolutely pure state and some impurities might be naturally occurring, thus giving a little added value to the crystalline over the synthetic. However, the *true vitamin* is the natural vitamin. So much for the quality of vitamins.

Now, when it comes to the right amount of vitamin and correct balance, it is always necessary to work with a professional. The exact amount of vitamins has to go hand in glove together with the right balance. The right balance should be established by a nutritionist who is specialized in vitamins. And then, yes, one can make *miracles* with vitamins.

MINERALS

The word *mineral* is derived from the word *mine*. Some minerals are also called *trace elements*, simply meaning chemical elements essential in a proper diet, but only in very small quantities. Just a *trace* is necessary. *Minerals* are inorganic substances (such as iron, needed by humans, animals and plants to stay alive), which occur naturally in the earth, hence the origin from the word *mine*. Some minerals are:

Calcium
Magnesium
Chloride
Iron
Potassium
Phosphorous
Chromium
Iodine
Copper
Manganese
Zinc.

One could write a whole book on minerals and vitamins. In fact, many thick books on the subject have been written. So, for practical purposes, we'll keep it short and sweet.

Without trace minerals, the body cannot manufacture or assimilate essential vitamins. A deficiency in magnesium and potassium would lead to damaged heart muscles. The body needs zinc and iron, among other minerals, for proper liver functioning. This is extremely important because your liver has the primary responsibility to cleanse your body of toxins, including drugs.

Not all trace elements are beneficial to one's health. Some of these are: lead, aluminum, cadmium and mercury. These are all toxic substances. If too many of these elements find their way into the tissues, the body will become ill and eventually die.

The big problem with minerals, like vitamins, is how to achieve a proper balance in the body. Have you ever heard the expression

"A little knowledge is a dangerous thing"? This is especially true when it comes to vitamins and minerals. Trying to apply incomplete knowledge can lead one in the wrong direction. Imbalances can be created in the body when one is trying to use vitamins and minerals to treat an illness. One may have been advised to take zinc to boost your immunity or to treat your chronic fatigue. This may be of some help but is not the whole answer by any means. Sometimes a quick improvement is mistaken for a cure. But if the beneficial effect is not long lasting, it is not a cure at all.

As with vitamins, the best mineral supplementation results are obtained when a good *natural* source is used. The body needs the right source and the right balance with micronutrients – vitamins and minerals – to restore and maintain its good health. It needs a good, ethical manufacturer and a professional nutritionist, and then vitamins and minerals are a true alternative to drugs.

But what if there are still drugs in the body? What if the body is so poisoned by environmental poisons and by medications that it is already sick. Is there a possibility to turn the cycle? To cleanse the body of old residuals from drugs and medication? Yes, there is. The following chapter probably contains the true secret for longevity.

But before we come to that, here's just one example in this interview (out of probably 100 possible techniques) to show what healing methods could be used instead of drugs.

DR. SHYLER NEVEAUX: "LIVING WITH CHRONIC PAIN IS AN OPTION NOT A NECESSITY"

Chinese medicine has been around for a very long time. In fact it is said to have originated 4000 years ago. That's a long time for a healing practice to survive. Many of the treatments are still being used to handle the ailments of the body today.

Just one example: the traditional herbal medicine. Chinese herbs are still being selected and combined in an organized fashion to affect various aspects of an illness in the same way that they did thousands of years ago. Use of these herbs is less likely to cause side effects than the correlated pharmaceutical drug because the complexity of the plant from which the herb comes causes it to be far more balanced than its counterpart drug which consists of isolated active ingredients.

Also included in Chinese medicine are acupuncture, dietary therapy, and exercises in breathing and movement called tai chi[336] and qi gong.[337] These have become popular among those who prefer to take up the more natural healing process. Dr. Shyler Neveaux is an expert in Chinese Medicine, having studied and even taught the subject at different universities.

"Tell us a little bit about your background first."

Dr. Shyler L. Neveaux, A.P., D.O.M., A.I.T.:[338] "I went to school for massage therapy in New York City, attending the Swedish Institute of Massage Therapy. This is the first school established for massage therapy in the country. It's

336 Tai chi: A Chinese system of meditative physical exercises used to improve and maintain good health, increase longevity and designed especially for self-defense and meditation

337 Qi gong: a Chinese system of combining breathing, mental focus, stretching, and movement to promote health, fitness, and relieve stress

338 A.P., D.O.M., A.I.T: Acupuncture Physician, Doctor of Oriental Medicine, Acupuncture Injection Therapist

been around for 60 years. There I studied western massage and shiatsu[339] for a year, and aced the test, by the way. Then I went to school for Chinese medicine."

"Where did you study Chinese medicine?"

Dr. Shyler L. Neveaux, AP: "I went to the Pacific Institute of Oriental Medicine in New York City and then graduated from the Florida Institute of traditional Chinese Medicine. After that, I attended the Texas State University for 2 years to become an acupuncture injections therapist."

"How about honors and awards?"

Dr. Shyler L. Neveaux, AP: "I hold an Acupuncture Injection Therapy Certification and a Laser Acupuncture Certification. As well, I have a certificate for the National Certification Commission for Acupunctures and Oriental Medicine. I am also certified in Homotoxicology[340]."

"Are you a member of any medical organizations?"

Dr. Shyler L. Neveaux, AP: "Yes. I am the member of the AAOM, which is the American Association of Oriental medicine. This is the oldest professional group there is. American Association of Oriental Medicine was formed in 1981 as the American Association of Acupuncture and Oriental Medicine. This was to be the unifying force for American acupuncturists who are committed to high ethical and educational standards. It is a well regulated profession that ensures the safety of the public."

---

339 Shiatsu: A form of therapeutic massage in which pressure is applied with the thumbs and palms to those areas of the body used in acupuncture

340 Homotoxicology: An approach that uses homeopathic remedies to rid the body of toxins that prevent its healing

"Do you give lectures?"

Dr. Shyler L. Neveaux, AP: "I actually give lectures all the time. Once a month I do a talk on fibromyalgia,[341] osteoporosis[342] and arthritis, but my favorite subjects are disc degeneration and spinal stenosis,[343] and arthritis in general. So far I have delivered over 30 lectures."

"How long have you worked with patients and how many patients have you treated?"

Dr. Shyler L. Neveaux, AP: "I have been in this practice for 8 years now and have treated approximately 4000 patients."

"About how many patients do you see in a week?"

Dr. Shyler L. Neveaux, AP: "I see about 30 – 50 patients in a week."

"What do you treat the most?"

Dr. Shyler L. Neveaux, AP: "I mainly treat pain. An example of this is my father. He had sciatica[344] and doctors said they couldn't do anything for him, but I was able to treat that in a pinch. His pain has diminished by quite a bit. I have also treated herniated and degeneration of the discs as well

---

341 Fibromyalgia: a syndrome characterized by chronic pain in the muscles and soft tissues surrounding joints, fatigue, and tenderness at specific sites in the body

342 Osteoporosis: a disease in which the bones become extremely porous, are subject to fracture, and heal slowly, occurring especially in women following menopause and often leading to curvature of the spine from vertebral collapse

343 Spinal stenosis is a narrowing or constriction of the passageway that the spinal cord goes through which results in pain

344 Sciatica: pain along the sciatic nerve usually caused by a herniated disk of the lumbar (of, near, or situated in the part of the back and sides between the lowest ribs and the pelvis) region of the spine and radiating to the buttocks and to the back of the thigh

as arthritis, osteoporosis, multiple sclerosis, Lou Gerigs disease,[345] Raynauds Syndrome[346] and even menopause and scleroderma."[347]

"Which therapy do you use that works best on the patient?"

Dr. Shyler L. Neveaux, AP: "That depends on the patient. Often we use acupuncture and homotoxicology together to detoxify patients. The best successes, of course, are based on patient compliance. We have a lot of success with handling pain. But first we would need to diagnose what is physically wrong with the patient."

"What is the best way to do this?"

Dr. Shyler L. Neveaux, AP: "We do this with an MRI Report. The MRI basically **is** the use of a special machine to produce electronic images of specific atoms and molecular structures, especially human cells, tissues, and organs. The scan of the human body will show if there is some abnormality present in that part of the body. Having found the abnormality, we can then begin the right treatment."

"Would you explain in simple terms what acupuncture is?"

---

345 Lou Gerigs disease is a chronic, progressive disease marked by gradual degeneration of the nerve cells in the central nervous system that control voluntary muscle movement. The disorder causes muscle weakness and atrophy and usually results in death.

346 Raynauds syndrome: a condition resulting in discoloration of the fingers and/or the toes after exposure to changes in temperature (cold or hot) or emotional events

347 Scleroderma: a pathological thickening and hardening of the skin and internal organs

Dr. Shyler L. Neveaux, AP: "Sure. The key word is balance – *homeostasis*.[348] In healthy bodies things are in balance. One can look at it as a triangle. The top part of the triangle is energy that is not flowing. This is called QI, which is the vital force thought to be inherent in all things as believed in by Taoism and other Chinese. The next one is blood stasis, which is blood not flowing, and the third part is organ imbalance. We have a system of channels on our body. Pain or discomfort means energy is not flowing in that area of the body so we move the energy, move blood and create an organ balance. This is what acupuncture does."

"Is there another way to describe acupuncture?"

Dr. Shyler L. Neveaux, AP: "Yes. Everyone has an ecosystem within his or her body. There are five elements at which we are looking. These are described in the old textbooks as 'wind, cold, dampness, dryness, and heat.' Acupuncture also balances this ecosystem within the body."

How is the balancing done?"

Dr. Shyler L. Neveaux, AP: "This balancing is done with fine needles applied to specific body areas which are pierced. This relieves certain body ailments. We also balance the ecosystem with acupuncture injection therapy."

"What is acupuncture injection therapy?"

Dr. Shyler L. Neveaux, AP: "This is the therapy where homeopathic substances are injected into the dermal layer at the pressure points. The injection stimulates the body to heal itself. Common homeopathic products that are used are *Arnica* and *Echinacea*. *Arnica* is used for muscle pain and

348 Homeostasis: the ability or tendency of an organism or cell to maintain internal equilibrium by adjusting its physiological processes

haematomas, which is when the flow of blood is forced from a vessel out into the surrounding tissue, while *Echinacea* is used to increase the natural defense system of the body."

"Is Chinese medicine really scientific?"

Dr. Shyler L. Neveaux, AP: "That is a good question, but please understand that Chinese medicine is 5000 years old. Modern scientific medicine is only 200 years old and therefore has not been put to the test, as has Chinese medicine. The word *science* has become so second rate that nearly anyone can attach it to their technology."

"Is there any proof that Chinese Medicine heals a person?"

Dr. Shyler L. Neveaux, AP: "The proof is within ourselves. No doctor can ever give us a hundred percent guarantee that he can heal someone. The body heals itself. Medicine is there only to support that healing."

"Have you seen it in the work that you do?"

Dr. Shyler L. Neveaux, AP: "Yes. In so many of the cases using Chinese medicine there is proof that it supports healing. I have seen it in the cases I work with. You could say that if it works, it must be right."

"Do you have any experience with pharmaceutical drugs?"

Dr. Shyler L. Neveaux, AP: "Yes. But first permit me to say this: Pharmaceutical drugs are the 4th leading cause of death in the country due to the side effects of the medication. I treat a lot of older people and there is always the fear of interaction with the medications they are taking. At the same time, they are afraid to stop taking the prescription they are on. In my opinion, side effects of drugs far outweigh the benefits of drugs. I get a lot of patients that are on medication of some sort, who are suffering from side effects."

"Give us an example of side effects you personally experienced with your patients?"

Dr. Shyler L. Neveaux, AP: "Well, okay, just one example. One of my patients developed fibromyalgia because of *Lipitor*[349] per her doctor. Side effects were aching, post-exertional fatigue, general malaise, chronic fatigue and bruises. One could say that many times the medication given to a patient will not work.

"Another example would be a 40-year-old woman who was in severe and constant pain for 12 months due to a pulled hamstring. She would experience pain from her low back down to her heel. This was due to a bulging disc, piriformis syndrome[350] and tendonitis[351] of her hamstring. The medication given to her by her doctor did not help and she could not sit comfortably during the day and woke up often all night due to pain. The doctor wanted to give her a *cortisone* injection, which would have been disastrous."

"Why is that?"

Dr. Shyler L. Neveaux, AP: "For one thing, the *cortisone* injection is not a permanent solution and it would erode the integrity of an already stressed joint. In other words, it would

---

349 *Lipitor* is used to lower cholesterol and triglyceride (fat-like substances) levels in the blood.

350 *Piriformis syndrome* is a condition in which the piriformis muscle irritates the sciatic nerve, causing pain in the buttocks and referring pain along the course of the sciatic nerve. Pain is known as sciatica.

351 *Tendonitis*: the inflammation of the tendon

have caused more damage. After only three treatments at our clinic, her pain was greatly reduced and after three months suffered only a mild discomfort when sitting too long."

"What did you use to treat her?"

Dr. Shyler L. Neveaux, AP: "What we used was acupuncture, cold laser,[352] injection therapy, and cross fiber friction[353] on her Ishial tuberosity.[354] This afforded her a healing and strengthening response approach without causing harm to the area."

"Have you actually enabled a patient to come off a drug after treating them?"

Dr. Shyler L. Neveaux, AP: "Yes. There was this patient with a heel spur.[355] The doctor had put her on *Vioxx*. We gave her one of the Chinese treatments called Lontophoresism where we apply an electrical current through a salt solution causing a migration of positive ions to a negative pole and radical ions to a positive pole. In this way excess calcium is removed and thus the pain is gone. After that she didn't need to be on *Vioxx. Vioxx,* you probably have noticed, has recently has recalled."

---

352 Cold laser: low energy lasers that penetrate deeply into the skin and work by improving metabolism, circulation and tissue healing

353 Cross fiber friction is massage that goes across the grain of the muscle in order to break down the adhesions between the parallel fibers within the muscle. This restores mobility and removes both toxins and deeply held patterns of tension.

354 *Ishial tuberosity*: the rough bony projection at the junction of the lower end of the body of the pelvic region

355 Heel spur is the more common name for plantar fascitiis. Plantar fasciitis refers to the inflammation of the plantar fascia (the tough, broad band of fibrous tissue located along the bottom surface of the foot that runs form the heel to the forefoot). Calcium deposits form when the plantar fascia pulls away from the heel area. This causes extreme pain.

"What is your opinion of pharmaceutical drugs and the big money?"

Dr. Shyler L. Neveaux, AP: "I have seen that the elderly take more drugs than other folks and they don't really handle anything. The pharmaceutical industry makes a lot of money off of the elderly."

"How about psychoactive drugs?"

Dr. Shyler L. Neveaux, AP: "I stay away from that. By using acupuncture, I can easily treat depression, and the patients' spirits soar. I had the experience of treating a friend with bipolar disorder.[356] She had these crying fits, but the drugs were not working for her. After acupuncture along with herbal formulas was applied, she no longer had these crying fits."

"Are there any other success stories you have in treating depression?"

Dr. Shyler L. Neveaux, AP: "Yes. Another female had been depressed for four years. She tried antidepressants but could not take the nausea, lack of sex drive and headaches. After her first acupuncture treatment, she said she was hooked. She felt elated, with a new outlook on life. The usual triggers that would stress her, and cause anxiety, and irritability no longer had such a strong influence over her. I put her on an herbal formula that relieves stress, and she is now doing very well."

"What is your attitude toward athletes and drugs?"

356 *Bipolar Disorder*: a psychiatric disorder marked by alternating episodes of mania and depression

Dr. Shyler L. Neveaux, AP: "I think that *Wobenzym*[357] is better than the steroid drugs."

"What is Wobenzym and what does it do?"

Dr. Shyler L. Neveaux, AP: "*Wobenzym* is a systemic[358] oral enzyme. It is an over-the-counter anti-inflammatory. *Wobenzym* normalizes the inflammatory response to injury or with any disorder that ends in 'itis,' which denotes inflammation. For example: arthritis, colitis, bronchitis, sinusitis, prostatitis, and pancreatitis."

"Where did Wobenzym come from?"

Dr. Shyler L. Neveaux, AP: "This product comes from Germany where it outsells *aspirin* for pain relief and inflammation reduction. Inflammation is the body's first response defense but it gets out of control, which is why *Vioxx* was so popular. Using *Wobenzym* controls inflammation and pain, enhances the immune system, and detoxifies the body."

"What technique do you use to get drugs out of the body?"

Dr. Shyler L. Neveaux, AP: "In our clinic, we have treatments to help people stop smoking which use acupuncture along with homotoxicology. In homotoxicology, we use several tinctures at the same time to detoxify the cellular matrix, and we use hormones, toxicology and herbs, as well."

---

357 *Wobenzym* is a combination of purified, naturally occurring enzymes that have proven to help control joint inflammation, improve healthy circulation, enhance immune function, and speed the recovery from strains and sprains. Enzymes are substances within the body that enable vitamins, minerals or hormones to do their jobs.

358 Systemic: relating to or affecting the entire body or an entire organism

"What successes have you had with the treatments?"

Dr. Shyler L. Neveaux, AP: "We had a guy come in a wheel chair who had experienced an accident in a plane. At the age of 41/42 years old, he was unable to defecate or urinate on his own and was sexually incapable. After massage and acupuncture he finally regained feeling in his legs and feet and can walk again. He defecates and urinates now on his own as well as experiences partial erections."

"Are there other successes?"

Dr. Shyler L. Neveaux, AP: "Another example is a nurse on the same flight who had severed arteries and swelling in her leg muscles and was in pain. The doctors had made cuts in her legs to reduce edema in the area. She had scars in her legs like purple angry ribbons. With treatment this has now improved and they can hardly be seen."

"Have you ever experienced treating a patient with such good results that saved her from a more drastic treatment from a medical practitioner?"

Dr. Shyler L. Neveaux, AP: "Oh, yes! One patient was being treated for Raynauds Syndrome or scleroderma and she developed a sore on her finger. The doctors were going to cut it off because of lack of circulation. However, with four acupuncture treatments she pinked up, was energetic and her appetite was better three-fold. She had a healing crisis. Her wound was healing and her doctor said to keep doing what she was doing, as she had never looked so good. She lost her fingernail but not her finger. Everything improved at work and with her granddaughter with whom she was having difficulty."

"Are there any other successes of this caliber?"

Dr. Shyler L. Neveaux, AP: "Yes. Another patient had a non-healing wound on the bottom of her foot. Doctors wanted to cut her foot off. Instead she was told to lose 100 pounds. By using the cold laser treatment, it took 8 months for sores to resolve, but she lost weight and they did resolve."

"How about successes with acupuncture injection therapy?"

Dr. Shyler L. Neveaux, AP: "We had this woman come in with sciatica and the doctors had wanted to give her a steroid injection (cortisone). She had compressed and bulging discs as well as a running injury in her hamstring. I saw her and told her to get rid of her high heels and gave her treatments. After the 2nd treatment she was 80% better. I used acupuncture injection, laser and magnetics, while she took glucosamine and enzymes for her discs. In the final analysis, she did not need the cortisone that would have destroyed her joint without even taking care of the problem."

"Do you have a motto?"

Dr. Shyler L. Neveaux, AP: "Yes. 'Living with chronic pain is an option, not a necessity.'"

11. FIGHTING DRUGS AND FINDING ALTERNATIVES (2): THE DIFFERENCE

When it comes to cleaning, cleansing and detoxification of the body, we face an entire tradition. In fact, there are literally hundreds of different detoxification programs in existence. Usually the purpose is to cleanse the body of old, harmful, toxic, unhealthy substances.

The earliest cleansing programs are probably the fasting techniques that have been known since at least four thousand years ago. We know fasting exists in Buddhism, in Hinduism and in Islam, and yes, in nearly all religions. In addition, today one can find all sorts of medical fasting procedures. In Europe, the most famous are the fasting techniques of Dr. Buchinger, the cleansing of the bowels by Dr. F. X. Mayr, and the so-called Dr. Schroth treatment. In the United States, one encounters other detoxification procedures and colon cleanser techniques. Often *clay* is used because it absorbs toxins in the intestine and "helps remove them from the body." [359]

Clay works like a magnet. Dr. Weston Price pointed out that primitive people in Central Africa and in Australia used clay as cleansing. Water has been used and was used in cleansing for centuries but only *healthy* spring water, since our tap water itself usually contains many toxins.

A breakthrough detoxification program was put together by L. Ron Hubbard[360] who developed the so-called *Purification Rundown.* ® Literally tens of thousands of success stories can be provided. The bad effects of old drugs, old medication can be undone. L. Ron Hubbard, in addition, was the only one who developed a complete technique to undo the partially horrible mental effects of drugs. Tons of success stories prove the workability of this ingenious technique.

---

359 Jordan S. Dubin, Joseph Brasco, *Restoring Your Digestive Health,* (New York, NY: Twin Streams, 2003), p. 194

360 L. Ron Hubbard, *Clear Body, Clear Mind,* (Los Angeles: Bridge Publications, 1990)

But again, this book is about *drugs*. The fact with cleansing is that we fight drugs, we fight the side effects of drugs, and therefore detoxification needs to be mentioned. Factually, detoxification is said to help in the healing process. The thousands of success stories that patients wrote cannot be ignored. So after nutrition is corrected, one should do a detoxification program. There are very sophisticated methods, just to clean the liver alone and possibly avoid or handle a host of diseases.[361] But our nutrition today is normally so depleted that we must not forget to talk about vitamins and minerals. Even today pharmaceutical drug companies sometimes produce vitamins. So here another surprise is waiting for us. But let's take a look at the last interview before we come to the final conclusion.

361 Dr. Sandra Dabot, *The Liver Cleansing Diet*, see www.liverdoctor.com

GERD SCHALLER: "EVEN THE PHARMACEUTICAL INDUSTRY ADMITS: THERE ARE NO DRUGS WITHOUT SIDE EFFECTS."

Gerd Schaller, born in 1944, German in origin, is known in many first-class companies as a top professional in relation to Direct Marketing techniques. Some of his clients read like the "Who's Who in Business Success" and belonged and belong to the upper tenth of the upper twentieth of economic prosperity.

But this frequently published author made a big change about five years ago. He started a completely new career in the health industry. Today, Gerd Schaller is the Executive Director of *Nature Power Trading Ltd.*, a company that has tens of thousands of customers. The company concentrates on nutritive supplements and is one of the key opinion leaders in the field of alternative healing in Great Britain. As well, the company increasingly provides those supplements to other countries.

Because of this international approach, we are able to obtain from Mr. Schaller a broader viewpoint to this problem called *drugs* and *side effects* than one normally does, because he has personally spoken to over 4000 people about this topic. Let's jump right into the subject.

"Mr. Schaller, what are your personal experiences with medical drugs? And what are your experiences with drugs in relation to your many customers?"

Gerd Schaller: "I guess my personal experiences are similar to other people's. Actually, I had to learn that nearly all of us have a history of different doctor-prescribed drugs. In the past, I thought doctors wanted to help. For example, I even thought an inoculation against influenza would be the perfect idea. I had to learn the hard way that inoculation is often a lie and only helps to fill the pockets of some pharmaceutical companies. After receiving a preventative inoculation against influenza at one point in my life, I came down with the flu like never before, and never after that. Later I obtained the information that the pharmaceutical industry often uses mercury – and they label it with very different scientific names to hide it – to preserve the vaccine over a long time. So personally, drugs hit me very badly.

"In addition, I know that some of our customers came down with multiple sclerosis a few days after an inoculation. They were not born with this disease.

In Germany, we have a situation wherein each newborn child gets its first inoculation a few days after birth. Actually, they just get their first dose of mercury.

"Women, already loaded with mercury, detoxify their bodies during pregnancy; they just transfer about 50% of their mercury via placenta to the foetus. The result that can be widely seen is a growing number of kids with neuro-dermatitis and ADHD. To put it simply, they have problems with their skin and problems in learning.

"But mercury is just one devil, although a dangerous one. Dentists use it as well. We have 82 million people living in Germany and 49 million of them have new inlays made out of amalgam per year. But mercury is present in amalgam. I must tell you, that in some countries like Sweden and even Russia, amalgam inlays are forbidden.

"This is only one of the problems that can be caused by drugs or substances used in medicine."

"Can you give other examples?"

Gerd Schaller: "Oh, I could give many. Some doctors, for example, prescribe antibiotics for virus infections – but everybody knows that they do nothing for viruses. Other doctors use it to fight bacteria – and they don't even bother to find out what bacteria is causing this particular illness; they just try a standard antibiotic and if it doesn't help, they try another one.

"However, antibiotics cause a lot of side effects, as well as ruin your intestinal flora. This is standard knowledge. I suppose that only a minority of the medical personnel prescribe a gut flora supplement to a patient who has taken antibiotics."

"What else?"

Gerd Schaller: "Oh, we have thousands of customers, and nearly all of them suffer from the side effects of medical drugs. Each of them was not able to find the necessary help to get rid of certain illnesses. There is hardly a customer who is satisfied about his past medical treatment. Most of them suffer inveterate diseases. I could give you a shockingly long list."

"So what` s wrong with the pharmaceutical industry today?"

Gerd Schaller: "The answer, in short, is that the pharmaceutical industry is often only interested in *curing* symptoms. If one has a headache, they have a pill or some drops to help him get rid of it quickly. They are very good at that. But they don't ask what really causes his headache. They don't have pills or drops to really handle the cause of his headache, which perhaps could even be caused by toxicities. Perhaps he drank too much beer, wine or other alcohol. They just give us a little red or white pill to conceal our pains and the real reasons behind them. We feel free of pain and instead of changing our lifestyle or undergo a detoxification we just go on. So we think the pharmaceutical industry has wonderful solutions. These companies are very successful with this method. Most of them are not really interested in healing. Why? It would ruin their business if they told us to detoxify instead of take a pill. From a business viewpoint, they are unable to stop their brand of selling drugs – and I can guarantee that they won't stop, ever."

"So what are the results? Please give a specific example."

Gerd Schaller: "In my opinion, each new pharmaceutical pill will increase the amount of poison in our bodies. They offer poison to obscure another poison. And if the red pill does not help, they give the patient a blue pill to handle the side effects of the red one.

"My father is 84 years old and suffering from Alzheimer. It could very well be that this disease is the result of toxicities caused by pharmaceutical pills – at least this is the theory of some researchers. My father has a long history of taking pills. Here in Germany, we have a situation that 30% of all people over 80 years of age suffer from dementia; it is unbelievable. But it is big business. No-one tells the truth about the causes, which I believe truly lie in several medical drugs (like certain heart attack medicines), heavy metals (especially aluminium and mercury), and a lack of vitamins, minerals and some amino acids. Alzheimer could probably be avoided if people would live more natural lives and consider a detoxification program occasionally. Currently my father has to take twenty different pills each day – with actually no hope that his health will ever come back."

"Who is responsible?"

Gerd Schaller: "We all are. Of course, Big Pharma is in the first place. But, in addition, the mighty doctors' associations, the food manufacturers and the consumers themselves are; we are talking about a huge lack of knowledge about natural health. It is easy for Big Pharma to sell drugs: we don't ask, we don't look; we just take the drugs, believing that it is much more convenient to take them instead of changing our habits. We allow them to carry on their big business by not opposing them. We allow them to take our money. This makes it easy for the pharmaceutical industry to present one pill after another, and we love it, because we are waiting for the next miracle pill."

"What is the exact mechanism behind it?"

Gerd Schaller: "Big Pharma tells us it is more important to fight against the one illness, and we have to agree that there are some side effects. Even the pharmaceutical industry itself admits there are no drugs without side effects. That is the price for our convenience. The doctor says, 'But you can get rid of your headache. Oh sorry, you might get gastritis, but we have solutions for that, too.'"

"What are the exact numbers in relation to failure?"

Gerd Schaller: "Each year in Germany about 40,000 people die because of the side effects of the medications from the pharmaceutical industry. In the USA about 200,000 a year."

"But what about the successes of the pharmaceutical industry? There is a lot of talk about anti-aging pills, prolonging of life, and new great inventions."

Gerd Schaller: "The facts are the facts, and the numbers are the numbers.

Here are some of those numbers: Of all 70-year-old Germans, 96% have at least one disease. Every third person over 70 years of age suffers from five or more illnesses simultaneously. More and more people, in Germany, in England and in the USA, need professional care when they get old; it is already a lucrative industry. Every third child and every fifth adult suffers from at least one allergy. In the year 1900, 15% of all men died because of heart/circulation diseases; today it is 50% in some countries.

"To make a long story short, I can't see any progress here. One also has to realize that some so-called scientific research papers are forged, or at least manipulated to a degree."

"What is the connection between money and the pharmaceutical industry?"

Gerd Schaller: "This connection is very obvious, isn't it? I just quote from Bayer's 2001 company report: 'Lipobay®/ Baycol® was said to be one of the growth boosters of the pharmaceutical industry. Having been on the market since 1997, the anti-cholesterolemic has become a *blockbuster* in no time; at last the turnover forecast was € 2.5 billion a year. Worldwide, approximately 6 million people were on the Bayer product. The decision of August 8, 2001 to take the product from the market, therefore, had extensive consequences for the whole group. *Vioxx* had an unbelievable sales share of 20% in the total turnover of the Merck & Co. group.'

"There are more than fifty years of medical and scientific progress between *Thalidomide* and *Vioxx*. Well, this is cynical, but what has really changed?

"Nevertheless, the pharmaceutical industry still has the nimbus of *scientific nature* and of *progress*, and those researching pharmaceutical companies justify their high prices with their high costs for research and development before these new medicinal products can finally be marketed to become a blockbuster. I don't need to comment on this any further, do I?"

"What about all those alternative companies?"

Gerd Schaller: "Indeed, there are thousands of small companies worldwide that devote themselves to naturopathy and truly endeavour to hold high the banner of natural remedies. However, they are faced with permanent pressure to prevent them from saying that the products from Mother Nature can *heal*. Worldwide it is a criminal act to claim that natural active substances – mainly ones from the body – can heal. Vitamin C as ascorbic acid can only be marketed in many countries in powder form in plastic containers. If it is filled into capsules, many countries considered it to be a medicinal product and hence needs a marketing authorization by law. That sounds unbelievable, but it is true.

"It is the law and one can be sentenced if it is violated. Naturopaths are being prosecuted – not because they cause harm – but because they violate laws that on the long term are intended to secure privileges for certain people and certain very big companies. And this is the privilege to have the right to control the health market at their own discretion, and to create *blockbusters*, explaining to us all the while that the chemical industry can heal our illnesses. Existing laws give them the right to disqualify the thousands-of-years old naturopathy as *unscientific*."

"Why don't our doctors protest?"

Gerd Schaller: "Because they are part of the system. As soon as a special medication is sanctioned to be on the market, the doctor can no longer do anything wrong – can he? He gave up his responsibility to the system.

"He now has the perfect insurance, in other words; everything is legal. He now has a so-called scientific permission to use this medication. We can no longer attack him; we cannot sue him.

"On the other hand, that same system can sue any doctor who is using a different approach. This system, consisting of the legal power of the government, big Pharma and the doctor's associations, watches like a hawk to ensure nothing changes. Every alternative approach is called *unscientific*. Every alternative research is suppressed. But the allegedly *scientific* research is published by an exact ritual."

"But there exists alternative research as well."

Gerd Schaller: "Yes. But funny enough it doesn't get published broadly. Additional new and very expensive research is asked for, which no one can pay. Research is delayed. The system owns enough money to stop alternative efforts."

"What would be a possible solution?"

Gerd Schaller: "I have daily contact with patients, doctors and pharmacists. Some know very well how this system works.

"Some of them have decided not to support this system any more. They look for alternatives. They leave Germany or other countries, and help people in countries that still permit them to heal and help people with solutions other than the so-called scientific solutions of the pharmaceutical industry. More and more people are in disagreement with these solutions; here develops a movement. *Freedom of therapy* is the slogan.

"Right now there aren't enough people who disagree. But the number of protesters grows. One day the old system will collapse from within. There are more and more doctors who suddenly realize their responsibility, and for whom integrity is more important than the dollar."

"What types of patients are already treated with alternative approaches?"

Gerd Schaller: "People who are chronically ill usually prefer alternative medicine. Most of them know that the side effects of the *system* are more dangerous than the disease they suffer from. In addition, most of them have been treated wrongly. There the phenomenon of wrong medication, over-medication and deadly medication exists."

"What is the first most efficient act the individual can do to escape the system?"

Gerd Schaller: "Every one of us can change nutrition. This is the true culprit of many dangerous diseases.

"For example, in East Germany, before the wall came down, approximately 10% of the population suffered from allergies. Since the wall came down, about 30% now suffers from allergies. Just after 15 years.

"The reason behind that is poor nutrition. People in East Germany today eat the same bad food as people in West Germany. There is only one logical consequence: we eat poorly. So we have to change our diet."

"To put it bluntly, in which direction should one change?"

Gerd Schaller: "One should avoid sugar in all its forms, also the hidden sugar in canned food and in beverages. It is, in any case, clear that one should not drink alcohol and not smoke. In addition, one should eat lots of fresh vegetables and fruits but of organic origin.

"And if one eats meat, eat organic meat only and not too much. In addition one should take vitamins and minerals, plus amino-acids and enzymes."

"What is the single most destructive influence of our times in relation to this topic?"

Gerd Schaller: "A very seductive question, but there is no single most destructive influence. However the culprits are the pharmaceutical pills themselves, the use of chemicals at home, heavy metals like aluminum, arsenic, cadmium, copper, lead, mercury and nickel, chemicals in our water, artificial stuff in our food, and of course street drugs and alcohol."

"In your opinion, what is the most effective way to make up for the damages we have done in the past to our bodies?"

Gerd Schaller: "One should undergo purification techniques. Today one can even purify the liver, the gall bladder and each individual organ.

"To cleanse the liver, it only costs $25, but a gall bladder operation costs perhaps $4000, or more. One can cleanse from parasites, fungi, heavy metals, and any old, illness-causing debris in our bodies. One can clean the gut, and it's important to know that our gut is 80% responsible for our immune system. One can clean the kidneys, and indeed the whole organism. Even modern technologies exist today that have special cleansing programs as in the case of Alzheimer.

"In fact, many diseases with impressive *scientific* names can be handled just by cleaning and purification techniques alone."

"Let's get a specific example here. What could one do in case of heart problems?"

Gerd Schaller: "Well, first of all, I am not a doctor and I cannot give any advice. And secondly, each patient is different. However, a more general advice would be: live a life that prevents the problem arising in the first place.

"In our industrial nations, heart problems are the number one cause of death. First of all, there are special risk factors like smoking, lack of movement and exercise, poor nutrition, lack of vitamins and minerals. Alcohol should be taboo, and cigarettes definitely. Here one must say "no."

"On the positive side, one can say that specials oils are important, such as cold-pressed olive oil for example. Antioxidants help, as do Vitamin C, E and Co-Enzyme Q10. In addition, Vitamin B12 and B6, Omega-3-fatty-acids, folic acid, Magnesium and L-carnitine (a special protein-building substance) are vital.

"Together with the right nutrition and exercise one can probably avoid heart-problems to an astonishing degree.

"However, even when the problem is already there, one can do a lot with the right nutrition and the right nutritive supplements; many people don't know how far this help can actually go."

"What about depression and fear? Here the doctors very quickly prescribe pills."

Gerd Schaller: "Unfortunately yes. But many folks don't know that even bad eating habits can cause depression. In addition, allergies may be responsible for depression if one continues to eat the wrong food. Even excessive coffee may be the culprit or too much sugar.

"On the other hand, Vitamin B1, B2, B3, B6 and B-Complex may help. Vitamin C is a must, as well as lecithin, calcium and magnesium. A lot of this advice can be found in literature, but Big Pharma is not necessarily interested in divulging this information.

"Sports and exercises are the third components in fighting depression naturally.

"When it comes to fear, again many people don't know that once more sugar may be the cowboy in the black hat. Special vitamins, calcium and magnesium are of utmost importance, as well. In general, of course, one has to ask a health-care specialist who is permitted to give advice and is knowledgeable in natural therapies."

"Now let's take up a really difficult subject like cancer. What can alternative medicine do in this case?"

Gerd Schaller: "This is a tricky subject, because when one talks about cancer one immediately faces opposition from the *system* as I call it. This much is true: many charlatans operate in this field – on both sides, by the way.

"First of all, one has to differentiate the many types of cancer. Some are not even very dangerous and are easy to heal today. But cancer is a shock word and it is used to impress people. Again prevention should be the talk of the day. General advice for every type of cancer is nearly impossible to give – there are too many forms. But if one would be forced to do so, one would give the advice to do all sorts of cleaning and cleansing methods – all sorts of purification first. In fact, complete packages of know-how exist today when it comes to cancer.

"One thing to note, the environment can cause cancer. We live today in a polluted world. Again, purification should be popular. Secondly, poor nutrition may be responsible. Special types of nutrition stop cancer from growing. On the other hand, certain nutrition can support cancer.

"Too much fat, especially animal fat and even cow-milk have been named as culprits; meat grilled or fried is worse than meat cooked. Stale fat, rancid oil, excessive sugar, bad carbohydrates, food with fungi in it, pesticides, artificial food colors, alcohol, coffee and even harmful chlorinated drinking water may contribute to cancer.

"Helpful nutrition for example would be: corn products, organic vegetables and fruits, salads, onion and garlic.
"In addition, antioxidants are important, as well as beta-carotene, vitamins, especially E and C and B complex; in fact nearly all Bs, B 12 and B17 are champions in helping in the case of cancer.

"However, there are entire books on this subject today, and my remarks should not be misunderstood as medical advice."

"So in a word there is a very different type of approach. How would you envision the health sector over the next 100 or 200 years?"

Gerd Schaller: "Well, permit me to give an extensive answer. Martin Luther King, the famous American pastor and civil rights leader once said, 'I have a dream.' He fought for the rights of the Afro-American community, and he won despite many obstacles. He fought against suppression and for social justice. He ended up in jail more than 30 times and many people tried to kill him.

"Basically he created a movement. Many people, black and white, shared his vision. His dream was that all people were equal in the eyes of the law, whatever color they have. He fought against racism and he fought for freedom. What did he do? He repeated the same message again and again, in hundreds of speeches and in many tractates.

"We have to do the same. There are many problems on this planet that have to be solved. One is the oil price. When the price for gasoline goes up, we just complain. The TV commentators talk about it a little bit, and tomorrow the topic is forgotten. And then we accept.

"But what would happen if we would just not agree? What would happen if the consumers would join together and all together say to one of those companies, 'No, we will no longer buy gasoline from you until the price is really low.'

"After awhile it would have to accept lower prices in order to avoid bankruptcy. Then one could take on the next oil company."

"So what is your dream?"

Gerd Schaller: "May I give a really long answer?"

"Please do."

Gerd Schaller: "I have a dream that our efforts join together to create a saner, better health industry.

"Man has started to intervene into the natural routine processes of life and is on the verge of destroying the natural order on our planet. We are destroying woods and inventing medicinal products which no longer cure but cause long-lasting damage to the well balanced harmony and function of our bodies.

"It is time to distinctly announce that health for all living beings can only be achieved if things are in line and in agreement with natural laws. By not curing the causes of illness but by merely fighting symptoms by interfering in body processes, and hence bringing about additional undesired side effects, pharmaceuticals have not, by any means, improved man's health during the past decades. There is a worldwide increase of illness, and man is buying a supposedly longer life expectancy at the price of a distinctly lower quality of life in one's old age. This is demonstrated in a dramatic increase of dementia and other diseases caused by today's lifestyle.

"I have a dream to show functional ways, in harmony with nature, which can be followed by everyone with or without therapeutic support in order to take back responsibility of one's own health into one's own hands.

"I have a dream to increase man's knowledge about successful healing techniques. He is the only one who is capable of making himself recover even if he sometimes depends on some good advice.

"I have a dream that not only the experts, but also everyone knows naturopathy, and that this precious knowledge will not become lost. Naturopathy – unlike arguments that occasionally come up – is by no means unscientific. Naturopathy can successfully treat on the basis of thousands of years of experience with naturopathic treatment.

"I have a dream we start re-thinking the true causes of illnesses and diseases more carefully, and listen again to the words of Prof. Dr. Antoine Béchamp, who said 'Le microbe, c`est rien, le milieu, c`est tout' – The microbe is nothing, the milieu is everything.

"I have a dream that people die less because of the side effects of pharmaceutical products.

"I have a dream the word *science* is not misused by the high priests of Big Pharma.

"I have a dream naturopathic healers are not threatened by the mighty pharmaceutical industry.

"I have a dream Big Pharma loses its privileges in relation to healing and the *system* is corrected.

"I have a dream naturopathic healers are not looked at as criminals in some countries.

"I have a dream everybody can choose the medicine and healing therapy he wants.

"I have a dream that the ministry of health is measured by the amount of people who are healthier than before.

"I have a dream that more and more responsible doctors see what is really going on and join the movement of naturopathic healing.

"I have a dream people recognize naturopathy as the oldest kind of medical science. It is neither *primitive* nor has it outdated itself, and even modern society is part of nature. It was back in the Stone Age when man discovered the healing benefit of various herbs. The ancient Greeks saw the first practicing and teaching physicians who were written into history books; long before that time there were shamans and druids. In the Middle Ages naturopathy was cultivated in monasteries.

"I have a dream people learn that illness is always a lack of something or that there is something in the body that should not be there.

"I have a dream that every one of us is free to choose the medical treatment that we have decided to be the right choice and method. In my dream, there are physicians who are free of the constraints of an institutionalized doctor's office and, with the mutual agreement of their patients, apply such therapy that they consider suitable for them; hence they will not be disciplined by or excluded from various organizations or associations.

"I have a dream that those politicians and secretaries of state responsible for the health resort are not judged by the political enforceability of higher contribution rates to health insurance companies but by what they have done to improve people's health in a measurable way and with a lasting influence.

"I have a dream we find ourselves in the end to have achieved real progress and not a pretended one. I am dreaming of the day when *medical progress* is not just a PR cliché but true reality. In my vision, better health resulted in decreasing costs for the health care system.

"I have a dream that we have a world where naturopathy without constraints and threats has the same liberties that our legislation has given to the pharmaceutical industry. In my dream, the better concept will be successful on a free market with no regulations, for the benefit of the individual and then for the benefit of all.

"I have a dream that health information is provided in a way everybody can understand. It is my dream, the usual medical mumbo-jumbo that the ordinary citizen cannot comprehend will be forbidden one day. I believe that it is urgently necessary to tell people the truth about the side effects of one method compared with another one in a much more compelling and lucid way.

"I have a dream more and more responsible doctors give up being afraid of losing income and reputation, and decide to show the people the way to long-term and natural health by means of proper nutrition.

"I dream of a time that can be compared to the past when doctors in China could become very rich because they succeeded in having an abundance of healthy patients. Such a doctor used to have a plethora of lanterns in front of his house so one could see that he was very successful and the people in his surroundings were very healthy. May all our doctors be wealthy and have many lanterns as long as they bring us health instead of medical products with side effects.

"I have a dream we unite many individuals into a huge movement. We are convinced that only a target-oriented unification of all those who are focused on natural health will bring about the achievement of permanent and effective positive changes.

"I have a dream we are free to make our own decisions. In my dream, there are more and more people each day who also make use of their liberties and thus contribute to make our dream of health come true in exactly the way we expressed it.

"I have a dream every one of us uses the freedom of speech and we unite in this noble cause."

"Mr. Schaller, thank you very much for sharing your vision with us."

12. FIGHTING DRUGS AND FINDING ALTERNATIVES (3): A WORD ABOUT HEART DISEASE AND CANCER

It would be a promising experiment to take all the major diseases and causes for death, which are in existence today and compare the drug treatment with that of alternative treatments.

One would be surprised.

Truth and nothing but truth is that some multi-billion drugs and their "treatments" don't heal at all. One could call that fraud, yes. We are not talking about side effects here any more we are talking about efficacy, pretended efficacy. However let us take a quick look on some *hot* subjects: cancer and heart problems, to prove our statement.

THE HEART DISEASE AND CANCER MYTH

According to the USA Department of Health and Human Services, "Heart disease and cancer continued to be the leading and second leading causes of death, together accounting for over half."[362]

Now, that is quite a statement to make in lieu of all the heart medications and cancer treatments that are on the market. And what a market that is! But before we go into the insidiousness of these medications and treatments, not to mention the covert marketing of these, let's look at some more statistics.

STATISTICS OF THE TOP KILLERS

The USA Department of Health and Human Services goes on to state that in 2002, in the United States, 28.5% of all deaths are due to heart disease and 22.8% due to malignant neoplasm, (which is cancer). This accounts for 51.3% of all deaths. One might then

362 National Vital Statistics Report for 2002, volume 53, Number 5, October 12, 2004 http://www.cdc.gov/nchs/data/nvsr/nvsr53/nvsr53_05acc.pdf

say that there is still 48.7% for death caused by other causes. Take another look at the statistics and we see that the next one in line is cerebrovascular diseases (diseases of or relating to the blood vessels that supply the brain, otherwise known as strokes), which accounts for 6.7%. The rest comes to even lesser percentages.

Doesn't this make one wonder if, somehow, heart disease and cancer is being created within the human species? Do animals suffer the same percentages of heart disease and cancer? We will answer these questions later in this chapter.

In the UK, statistics state "diseases of the heart and circulatory system (cardiovascular[363] disease or CVD) are the main cause of death in the UK: accounting for just under 238,000 deaths in 2002. More than one in three people (39%) die from CVD."[364] It is easy to see that the USA is not the only country to have this problem. Well, what underlies this problem called heart disease and cancer? Let's take a look at what the heart diseases are first and cover cancer and its horror story later in the chapter.

TYPES OF HEART DISEASES

Heart disease can be divided into four types. The first is coronary artery disease. This is where the arteries become clogged and narrowed with fatty deposits (plaque), reducing blood flow to the heart muscle and causing chest pain (angina).

The second is heart rhythm problems, which is primarily an electrical conduction problem. It is an electrical impulse that causes the heart to beat in the first place and when this is disrupted, such physical difficulties such as palpitations, dizziness or weakness, and fainting occurs. This is because there is not enough blood being moved through the body.

---

363 Cardiovascular means of, relating to, or involving the heart and the blood vessels

364 Sophie Petersen, Viv Peto and Mike Rayner, "Coronary Heart disease statistics," 2004 edition, British Heart Foundation Health Promotion Research Group, Department of Public Health, University of Oxford http://www.heartstats.org/uploads/documents%5c2004pdf.pdf

Heart valve disease is the third disease and is the condition of a valve leaking in the heart causing a heart murmur. The heart has several valves that prevent the blood from moving backwards in the chambers within the heart and when the valve becomes faulty through disease, the blood slips back through the valve the wrong way.

Lastly, but not the least important, is heart failure. The heart just stops beating. There are three causes for heart failure. One is the well-known and feared heart attack in which the coronary arteries, through which the blood flows to the heart, are suddenly blocked by a ruptured plaque sac. The next cause is high blood pressure, which causes the heart to enlarge, and puts added stress to the heart muscle. Lastly, the heart muscle may become diseased itself causing the heart to become enlarged and inefficient.

There are various ways of treating these heart diseases, from using drugs to surgery. And then there are natural drug-free ways to prevent heart disease in the first place and to correct a faulty heart. Let's take a look at the various drugs that are currently used to treat heart diseases and leave the more natural treatments to the last.

HEART DISEASE MEDICATIONS AND THEIR SIDE EFFECTS

Usually when someone begins to experience the various symptoms of heart disease, they go see their family doctor. Of course! Heart failure has the reputation of being rather final in one's life. And because the doctor has invested interest in the pharmaceutical industry, he will prescribe medication. After all, what could be scarier than heart failure? The patient, now on medication, feels he has nothing to fear. Or is this true?

One might begin to wonder about the patient's security when one takes a look at the various side effects that these various drugs have.

Let's take the case of Coronary Artery Disease. In this case, deposits of fatty deposits block the arteries. Eventually, one of the plaque sacs ruptures and the blood clotting mechanism begins, forming a blood clot that travels to the heart and blocks the blood flow. Now a heart attack takes place. There are various drugs that are given to ease this condition. But note what the People's Medical Society has to say: "none of the drugs permanently clean up the narrowed areas and make things right again. Instead, they artificially alter the physiological situation and ease the heart's work."[365] These artificial methods vary. The doctor can widen the blood vessels or slow down the heart by use of drugs to reduce blood pressure. Or the patient can undergo surgery (which we are not covering at this point).

All the drugs prescribed for heart disease have side effects. Take *Coumadin*, for example. It thins the blood by blocking the coagulating action of the blood cells. Very nice, one might think, since it is the blood clots forming in the plaque-clogged artery that causes the heart attack in the first place. But look again. The clotting of the blood is one of the body's natural functions. Without clotting, a body can bleed to death. And yes, that is the main side effect of *Coumadin*. A person can bleed to death. I haven't even mentioned any of the other side effects such as cold intolerance, loss of appetite, stomach pain or cramping. And then the more infrequent side effects which sound even more horrifying such as gangrene, difficulty breathing, painful red sores, hives, fever, painful urination, jaundice and others too numerous to list here. I have seen elderly folks covered with bruises while they were taking *Coumadin* and it's not caused by bumping into things or being beat up. What are the doctors doing here? Playing with fire?

And this is not the only drug with such nasty side effects.

An over-the-counter drug, *aspirin*, is becoming more and more commonly promoted by the pharmaceutical companies and patients are taking a low dosage every day or so. *Aspirin* works like *Coumadin* in that it prevents clotting. Again, the same problem with bleeding occurs here as well as other side effects such as

365 *Your Heart: Questions you have... Answers you need*, (Allentown, PA: People's Medical Society, 1996) p. 69

kidney disorder after prolonged use, ulcers, brain hemorrhages, stomach pain, and asthma attacks if one is allergic to *aspirin*.

Particularly, in the case of brain hemorrhages, it may be well to note that Doctor Charles H. Hennekens, as the head of the 1988 "Physician's Health Study" (a study of *aspirin* use to prevent heart attacks) and a writer in the 1997 article, "*Aspirin* as a Therapeutic Agent in Cardiovascular Disease," stated "the findings for stroke as well as overall cardiovascular mortality were inconclusive due to inadequate numbers of events, but there was evidence of a possible increase in hemorrhagic strokes in the *aspirin* group." He goes on to say, "Although this finding was not statistically significant, any agent that inhibits platelet aggregation may pose a risk of increased bleeding."[366]

Heparin is another drug used as a blood thinner to prevent and treat blood clots, but it is labeled America's riskiest drugs. Getting the correct dosage is tricky and if the patient is given too much, he bleeds to death. Given too little would cause a blood clot to form, which, in itself, leads to a heart attack or stroke. But there are other side effects as well such as stomach pain or swelling, backaches, constipation, coughing up blood, headaches, fast breathing, hives, troubled breathing, skin bruising, and severe liver disease, among a list of many other symptoms.

Other drugs, which are used to control the production of cholesterol, are the *Statin* drugs. However, like *Coumadin* and a*spirin*, it has side effects too. And one that cannot be ignored is possible liver damage, which can develop without causing symptoms. The patient would never know that his liver was being damaged. Thus, when taking a *Statin* drug, the patient "should have their liver function tested periodically."[367]

Ace inhibitors reduce the deposition of plaque within the arteries and reduce the production of the hormone angiotension-2, which is

---

366 "Aspirin as a Therapeutic Agent in Cardiovascular Disease"; Charles H. Hennekens, MD; Mark L. Dyken, MD; ; Valentin Fuster, MD, American Heart Association, Inc. 1997, p. 1, http://circ.ahajournals.org/cgi/content/full/96/8/2751#R18

367 http://www.medicinenet.com/drug_induced_liver_disease/page8.htm

the hormone that triggers plaque rupture. Sounds good until one finds out that Ace inhibitors can interfere with kidney function.

Beta-blockers also reduce the plaque deposition. But a person can experience fatigue, worsened conditions of asthma, high blood sugar levels, and impotence. What a trade off! Newer beta-blockers have been developed which, the pharmaceutical companies have stated, do not cause these side effects. But if one views the track record for these companies, wouldn't it make him wonder what new side effects will show up after usage of these newer drugs over time?

It seems that in any of these treatments, one is opening a Pandora 's Box of other ills.

There is another concern that should be taken into account. This is the fact that the older generations, who are most set up for heart attacks, are already on various medications for other ills. This sets the scene for harmful drug interactions. For example, *Coumadin* should not be mixed with other drugs such as "sulfa" antibiotics (*Bactrim* and *Septra*) because of the risk of serious bleeding. *Aspirin* and *Ibuprofen* (a pain killer) taken with ACE inhibitors can decrease the effectiveness of the ACE inhibitors. *Viagra*, *Levitra*, and *Cialis* interact with the nitrate-based drugs to produce a sudden drop in blood pressure.

The Harvard Health Letter states, "The FDA maintains a thorough system for reporting drugs' side effects but currently lack a standardized method for warning people about drug interaction. This is largely due to the uncertainty and ambiguity surrounding this issue."[368]

Doesn't sound too encouraging. Perhaps the prevention is much more palatable than the cure, but we will take a look at that toward the end of the article.

368 http://www.newswise.com/p/articles/view/503846/ "The Harvard Health Letter" released Mar 2004

HORRORS OF CANCER TREATMENTS

Let's take a look at the treatment of cancer, the other main cause of death. Cancer is a group of diseases in which cells of the body grow, change, and multiply out of control. Various things can cause cancer and these are called carcinogens.

The various treatments today are surgery, chemotherapy, and radiation. There are studies to determine if *Angiogenesis*[369] *inhibitors* could possibly be a safe cure for cancer. These drugs "inhibit the formation of new blood vessels, causing the cancer to shrink and die. Whether Angiogenesis inhibitors will be effective against cancer in humans is not yet known."[370] So it is yet to be seen what these drugs will bring on as far as side effects go. However, let's look into the side effects of these other treatments.

Surgery is the cutting out of the cancerous cells. Although surgery is definitely a possible solution when it comes to removing small sites of cancer as in the case of skin cancer, the removal of larger cancerous sites poses a problem of its own and we will not take it up here. What we want to discuss, instead, is the side effects of chemotherapy and radiation, the two treatments that are used extensively to treat cancer.

Chemotherapy is the use of certain drugs that destroy the cancer cells and keep them from growing or multiplying. Sounds great! But what about the healthy cells? Do these drugs keep them from growing also? The answer is it does. And this can pose a problem if certain vitally needed cells are also destroyed. When these healthy cells are destroyed, there are side effects such as the temporary decrease in the number of white, red, and platelet blood cells causing increased risk of infection, anemia, and bleeding. There is hair loss on the head and body not to mention nausea, diarrhea,

---

369 Angiogenesis means the formation of new blood vessels. Angiogenesis inhibitors are drugs that blocks angiogenesis in cancerous tissue, thus interfering with tumor growth or metastasis.

370 "Angiogenesis Inhibitors in the Treatment of Cancer"; National Cancer Institute©; 2002 http://www.cancer.gov/cancertopics/factsheet/Therapy/angiogenesis-inhibitors

and vomiting. Some of the drugs used can cause heart and kidney damage. Not a pretty sight.

And what about radiation? Is this any better? First let's examine what radiation therapy is and then take a look at its side effects.

Radiation therapy uses a certain kind of radiation to kill cancer cells and shrink tumors. This radiation "injures or destroys cells in the area being treated (the "target tissue") by damaging their genetic material, making it impossible for these cells to continue to grow and divide."[371] Mind you, the radiation does not differentiate between healthy cells and cancerous ones, and this leads to side effects, also. These can be nausea, hair-loss, fatigue, low blood count or more serious ones like leukemia due to bone marrow cells being damaged from the therapy. Radiation also suppresses the immune system so that the patient can become sick with other diseases. But this is the price one pays when one gets cancer. Or is it?

Can it be that the pharmaceutical company, once again, has found another market from which to make its wealth? Is there an alternative approach to the handling of heart disease and cancer? Or do we have to settle for these side effects?

ALTERNATIVE APPROACH FOR HANDLING CARDIOVASCULAR DISEASE AND CANCER

Let's take a look at heart disease first. The major problem causing heart disease seems to be the deposit of plaque in the arteries, which constricts the flow of blood to the heart. So, one would think that the cure would be to get rid of the plaque and the prevention is to provide an environment whereby the plaque does not accumulate. Makes sense.

However, listen to what Dr. Rath has to say about cholesterol and plaque buildup. He says: "High blood cholesterol can lead to cardiovascular deposits only when combined with the loss of the integrity and functional weakness of the blood vessel wall, which

371 "Cancer Facts": National Cancer Institute©: 2004

triggers the need for its biological repair."[372] What an interesting concept! In his studies and writing, Dr. Rath claims that the pharmaceutical companies have told the doctors that it is the high cholesterol that is to blame. But is it? Is this just another marketing story of the pharmaceutical industry?

As we mentioned earlier in this chapter, animals do not have cardiovascular disease. And bears, for example, have a lot of cholesterol in their blood. Dr. Rath says in his article that animals manufacture their own vitamin C, whereas the human does not. It is the vitamin C that produces collagen in the body. Collagens are the reinforcement molecules of our body that provide stability for our blood vessel walls. With enough vitamin C, the human body would have fewer cases of heart attack.

Such a simple solution to preventing heart attacks. Build a healthy heart and blood vessels through exercise, vitamins and healthy life style. The book, "The 10% Solution for a Healthy Life"[373] by Raymond Kurzweil, tells how one can eliminate risk of heart disease and cancer. He goes over health issues such as smoking, taking drugs and alcohol, drinking beverages with caffeine, lack of exercise, and eating a high-fat diet. All of these contribute to the problems we have with heart disease and cancer.

Mind you, there are occasions where the taking of a drug is necessary, such as the life-and-death situation of a heart attack. Using under-the-tongue preparations of nitroglycerin at this time is known to prevent an angina attack by dilating the arteries. But here we are not talking about a long-term usage of the drug and so the side effects are negligible if there are any at all. Here we are talking about a life or death emergency.

So now we see that even with cancer, there is a natural way to prevent this insidious disease. But how about curing cancer? Can this be done without radiation, surgery, and chemotherapy?

---

372 "Cellular Medicine in Heart Disease", http://www.drrathresearch.org/lab_research/heart_disease.html

373 Raymond Kurzweil, *The 10% Solution for a Healthy Life*, (New York: Crown Publishers, Inc, 1993)

There are many different treatments for cancer that do not require surgery, chemotherapy, or radiation. Walter Last lists these in "The Diversity of Natural Cancer Cures."[374] The treatments range from natural raw food diets to use of special machines to kill the cancer cells, from special herbs and teas to ozone therapy. Many of these proved to be many times more effective with better remission (the period during which the symptoms of a disease abate or subside). And yet, as we read this article, we see that the Medical Association banned many of the possibly successful treatments. Today a person can be fined by even using the word "cure" in their therapies in regards to cancer. Makes a person wonder, doesn't it?

IN CONCLUSION

To conclude this treatise on heart disease and cancer, we see fit to make some conclusions on their treatments. It appears once again, that the pharmaceutical companies have found a target group for more experimentation, more lab work, and newer drugs to try out on the unsuspecting patient. All of this means more financial support, more funds from the government, and more money being spent by heart and cancer patients. For what reason? Why to line the pockets of the pharmaceutical companies, of course.

It is dubious that the life span of the patient in either case lives a longer life as a result of taking these drugs. In a recent magazine called "Der Spiegel,"[375] an epidemiologist states (after having made a discovery when he analyzed the rates of survival), "Despite all alleged progress, all sick people do not live one day longer." He goes on to say that "patients die as fast as they did 25 years ago." In fact, 100,000 die each year in Germany from cancer alone. This is astronomically high and expensive when it comes to the cost of medication. And on top of that, certain chemotherapeutical medicines killed a lot of patients inside

374 http://www.health-science-spirit.com/cancerdiversity.html

375 *Der Spiegel:* 41/2004 p. 160

a few weeks causing the medicine to be taken off the market. Astonishing and troubling! But what would one expect when it comes to the pharmaceutical industries that are mainly interested in making big bucks?

So we see that even with drugs, a person doesn't actually live longer. And even if so, what quality of life would he have with all these side effects plaguing him? Gives a person cause to question what the pharmaceutical companies are actually up to, doesn't it?

Now one could take up one subject after the other and we would be surprised. Prostate? Yes, a person can buy expensive drugs against prostate problems. And yes, he would have a good chance to suffer side effects. But instead, he could also increase his intake of zinc, really get into vitamins and minerals, use old Indian remedies (like saw palmetto), take pygeum africanum,[376] take up an intensive study of alternative medicines, find out the healing aspects of ginseng, bee pollen, special amino acids and even reduce the growth of the prostate and escape the problematic drugs and surgery. Of course, he would have to change his diet to an anti-prostate growing diet, which exists, as a matter of fact.

Chronic fatigue: yes, a person can try to handle the emotions that accompany it (fear, grief, a feeling of death) with Prozac, and, yes, he will have horrible side effects. Or he can study alternative medicines and find out again and again how important vitamins and minerals are, find out about immune enhancers, find out about Echinacea, suma[377] and other herbs like Paullina cupana,[378] gingko

376 Pygeum africanum: a tall evergreen tree from which tea is made from its bark to control urinary disorders in men

377 Suma: a South American herb used to help regulate and enhance your endocrine, nervous, digestive, cardiovascular and immune systems.

378 Paullinia cupana: an herb harvested from the Amazon rain forests, used to support mental alertness and fight fatigue.

biloba,[379] the wild yam, special proteins, enzymes like Q10[380] and escape doubtful medication therapies, with better effects often or at least sometimes.[381]

Do we say that alternative methods are always better and better working than the drug-oriented culture? Of course not. There are charlatans on both sides, and there are experts on both sides. Basically neutral, objective comparisons are missing.

However, this book is about the side effects of drugs, not about the alternatives. We only mentioned the other side, because it would be wrong to talk only about the negativity of something. Alternative experts have written quite a number of books – wonderful books. And we must not forget to mention chiropractors, nutritionists and alternative healers, who can inform you. The difference is this: natural medicines, which can't be patented, do not hold an interest for the pharmaceutical drug cartel. Why? No money can be made from them, or at least not enough money; it requires synthetics to patent something. A substance found in nature can't be patented. There is a wealth of data in relation to natural methods of healing.

So we don't have to move in the direction of a drug society. We don't have to be drug personalities to become healthy again. So what is the final conclusion?

379 Ginkgo biloba: derived from the leaves of the Ginkgo biloba tree, and used to treat blood flow disorders, mental decline (dementia), memory and concentration problems, asthma and allergies

380 Q10: a coenzyme useful as a heart disease remedy and as a treatment for a host of other ailments including cancer

381 Amazing Medicines, ibid. p. 104 and 135

13. THE FUTURE OF A DRUG-FREE SOCIETY

The circle comes to a full end. This book has proven all the statements we said in the first chapter. To reiterate here: Yes, we are praying to a new deity these days, and this God is called *drug*. Yes, we are made into believers of new religion – the drug religion. Yes, with drugs, we believe we can solve every problem. Thus say the drug pushers. Thus say the pharmaceutical industries.

But the real truth is that we are creating a population with less self-responsibility, with less responsibility for others. We are creating new diseases, which will, in turn, be fought by new drugs. Yes, we are moving into the direction of a DRUG SOCIETY.

Psychoactive drugs probably have the most horrible side effects. They can turn people into zombies making them less able to work and even lead to suicide. Drugs lead to higher welfare costs, an endangered older population and endangered children. We have actors and actresses on drugs, athletes on drugs, middle-age people on drugs and every other target-market a PR-mind of the big drug companies can think of. So the hidden Agenda of the pharmaceutical drug companies is to get us *all* on drugs. This way, DRUG PERSONALITIES are created. Simply, side effects and side effect of side effects are already the case. We even create our own new diseases of tomorrow.

Must this happen necessarily? Of course not! The wheel can be turned backwards, always. As well as envisioning a three-stage scenario, which point in the direction of a dying society, one can also postulate a three-stage scenario pointing to a new, alive, happy drug-free society. These three steps have to be taken if this world shall not be doomed:

STAGE ONE: What is needed is a combined effort to fight the criminal behavior of drug companies wherever possible. Partially this is already case. While this book is being written, *the Wall Street Journal* (Nov. 1. 2004) headlined: “EMAILS SUGGEST MERCK KNEW VIOXX’S DANGER AT EARLY STAGE.”

To quote the authors Anna Wilde Mathews and Barbara Martinez exactly: "...internal Merck e-mails and marketing material as well as interviews with outside scientists show that the company fought forcefully for years to keep safety concerns from destroying the drug's commercial prospects."

Let's take a last look at that never-ending story about *Vioxx*, a nice word, perhaps taking from the Latin root via which means life, while it is taking life, not giving? Well, this seems to be established at the time of this writing: nearly every hundred patients, says the Spiegel once upon a time taking Vioxx, (only after taking it one year) suffered a stroke or a heart attack. The real scandal? Those facts were known, per the Spiegel, before Vioxx was offered in 1999 to the market.[382] Emails have been found, emails within Big Pharma giant Merck, which prove that.

In Germany and in the USA, thousands of patients *sued* Merck.[383] Billions of dollars were at stake.[384] Finally, finally, after the smoke disappeared, it was established without doubt or reservations that this medication had caused stroke and heart attacks. An amount of 4.85 billion dollars had to be paid to 47,000 plaintiffs.

When do we begin to understand that it is not a single medication that is dangerous but the whole philosophy behind it, suggesting we could handle everything with a pill?

Despite early evidence of the danger of this medicine, the strategy of the Pharma giant consisted of calming down doctors who reported "bad news." Doctors who could be bought with money had to give lectures about how safe *Vioxx* was. [385] True data was suppressed by all means.

And the pharmaceutical industry itself?

Well, well! Very quickly a new medication from another pharmaceutical giant saw the light of this world. A new medication substituted the old one. *Arcoxia* is the name, slogan: power, vigor,

---

382 Spiegel 39/2005

383 Spiegel 6/2005

384 Spiegel 8/2005

385 Spiegel 46/2004

which moves. Perhaps the word *Arcoxia* is taken from the Latin root *arca* meaning bridge (arc) to show the strengths of this medication. But don't forget, *arca* can also mean jail and coffin, just another meaning of the Latin word. The Spiegel already asked if *Arcoxia* could also create heart attacks. [386]

However, we even don't want to go into detail here, because that is just *one* fight. But we are not prophets stating that more and more scandals will see the light of day. Too many side effects of side effects are possible. Brave men and women, courageous men and women, not corruptible, honest, the best of us, will report on those scandals. These brave people will not bow down in front of money and will not be impressed by multi-billion-dollar figures. They will see the future of the society at large, and will see responsibility when it comes to old and young people. Partially, we already see some courageous people fight this impossible fight and dream this impossible dream of a drug-free society.

Soon politicians will get involved, and while today many politicians are "sponsored" (we know a better word) by the pharmaceutical drug companies, there will come the time when truly responsible politicians will name the game and say what it is: drugs are destroying the health of many of us whilst filling the money-bag of a few of us.

Stage one will include that politicians in the future be forbidden to take *any* money from the pharmaceutical industry by law. People will no longer elect politicians who are linked to Big Pharma, and, despite all of the money in the world, those types of politicians will lose. More important, there will be politicians who see clearly what is going on and who will have the courage to act against the pharmaceutical fraud. They will be the last freedom fighters, and if this planet has any chance to avoid sinking in the mud of a drug-society, it will be because of those freedom fighters. But even courageous lawyers will see the just case more and more, independent judges will open their mouth and whole populations will not only ask for money if one of their beloved ones died but

386 Spiegel 7/2005

will ask to stop this whole destructive course. Bribery will be more and more the matter of court-cases and the fine will be higher and higher.

STAGE TWO will be the next step: There will be legislation against those new types of drug-barons, who, under a legal outfit, are drugging the society at large. Researchers, doctors, drug-professors will go to jail for murder, to say nothing of the pharmaceutical industry bosses. The pharmaceutical industry will shrink back to the place it should have which is about 0.01 of the size it has today. Alternative medicine will be the talk of the day, and false advertising will be illegal.Honest science will arise; psychiatrists will be recognized for what they are: pretending to be scientists while they are criminals in many cases. Psychiatry will be gone one day because of their own crimes and incompetence, which is so well documented throughout history. We will have strong anti-drug-movements as we had anti-war-movements, which will watch every little move those drug-companies do. Their true goal: money, money and money will be revealed. The stocks of these giants will fall. The rats will flee the sinking ship and public opinion will turn against the pharmaceutical drug cartel, which is hiding so perfectly up to today.

STAGE THREE describes a drug free society. Detoxification-programs will be the talk of the day, natural healing methods, vitamins, minerals, enzymes, plant-based cures and the host of the many other alternative medicines, which are already in existence. We will have 100% drug-free personalities, not on any medication, even when they are 90 years old. The environment will be cleaned bit by bit from chemical poisoning. We will have dine-in restaurants and fast-food drive-through restaurants who deliver whole foods instead of toxic, fattening foods. We will regain our original personalities, not doped and manipulated in whatever artificial emotion or attitude. Suicide will be less, better relationships will be possible, and the obsessive promotion of sex will be gone. We will have better families, higher IQs and a safe environment.

A paradise? A little one, yes. But the full truth is, every one of us decides in what direction we move. Every one has to make up his mind. And every one can talk, influence and fight.

There is no greater power than the single individual once he has recognized the truth.

Bibliography and Notes

Chapter 1:

1. In 2007, the manufacturers of vaccine have leaned more away from the use of mercury in their products.
2. USA General Accounting Office. *Report to the Chairman, Subcommittee on Human Resources and Intergovernmental Relations, Committee on Government Operations, House of Representatives: FDA Drug Review Postapproval Risks 1976-85.* Washington, DC: USA General Accounting Office; 1990:3.
3. http://www.brwwellness.com/three.htm
4. Parkinson's disease: a brain disease that causes tremor and makes muscles rigid
5. Quoted from http://www.brwwellness.com/three.htm
6. http://www.yourhealthbase.com/database/a78d.htm

Chapter 2:

7. Center for Policy Alternatives, "Playing Fair: State Action to Lower Prescription Prices," 2000
8. Public Citizen Congress Watch, "2002 Drug Industry Profits: Hefty Pharmaceutical Company Margins Dwarf Other Industries," June 2003 (www.citizen.org/documents/Pharma_Report.pdf). The data is drawn mainly from the Fortune 500 lists in *Fortune,* April 7, 2003, and April 5, 2004, and drug company annual reports.
9. See Kurt Langbein, Bert Ehgartner, Das Medizin Kartell (München: Piper, 2002).
10. Roy Porter, *The Greatest Benefits to Mankind,* (New York: W. W. Norton & Company, 1998)
11. http://www.chemheritage.org/EducationalServices/pharm/asp/asp180.htm
12. See Bayer AG-Company history 1881 – 1914 – http://www.bayeraspirin.com/pain/asp_history.htm

13. Infarction: an area of dead or dying tissue due to insufficient blood supply
14. DM: deutsche mark, German money
15. See http://www.bayeraspirin.com/pain/asp_history.htm
16. See http://www.bayeraspirin.com/pain/asp_history.htm
17. http://www.consumeraffairs.com/news04/2005/aspirin_skin_cancer.html
18. Wikipedia, http://en.wikipedia.org/wiki/Viagra
19. Recreational Drug Information, http://www.alb2c3.com/drugs/viagfaq.htm
20. Mike Hall, America At Work, http://www.aflcio.org/aboutaflcio/magazine/0503_bigfix.cfm
21. American Medical Network "Cialis Could Top Viagra by 2006." September 2, 2004. http://www.health.am/ab/more1/cialis_could_top_viagra_sales_by_2006
22. Ibid.
23. Center for Drug Evaluation and Research, Federal Drug Administration http://www.fda.gov/cder/consumerinfo/viagra/viagrafaq.htm
24. See Langbein, p. 85
25. Lipitor is used to lower your cholesterol. *Cholesterol* is thought to be the cause of hardening the arteries and so a cause of heart-problems.
26. *Norvasc* is used to treat high blood pressure. It is also used to treat a type of chest pain called *angina. Angina* is often a pain or pressure in the chest that keeps coming back when part of the heart does not get enough blood.
27. *Zoloft* allegedly treats depression and panic.
28. *Paxil* treats social anxiety disorder, depression and panic disorder.
29. *Augmentin* is an antibiotic in the class of drugs called penicillin.
30. *Flovent* aids in preventing asthma symptoms before they start.
31. *Zocor* blocks the production of cholesterol (a type of fat) in the body.

32. *Vioxx* is used to relieve the pain and inflammation caused by osteoarthritis. It is also used to relieve minor pain, headache, and menstrual pain and discomfort.
33. *Cozaar* is used to treat high blood pressure. It blocks the action of certain chemicals that tighten the blood vessels, so blood flows more smoothly.
34. See *Pharmaceutical Executive*, May 2002, pp. 62, 63.
35. "Top 50 pharmaceutical companies," MedAdNews, September 2007
36. Der Spiegel 15/2005, p. 86
37. *Zocor* is used to reduce the total amounts of LDL (bad) cholesterol, triglycerides (another type of fat) and apolipoprotein B (a protein needed to make cholesterol) in the blood.
38. "Profiting from Pain," *Families USA*, p. 5
39. See Uffe Ravnskov, MD. PhD, independent research, Spo, www.opinions3.com/Uffe_Ravnskov_Report.htm
40. http://bmj.com/cgi/content/full/324/7342/886
41. http://www.brojon.org/frontpage/SARSFEVER.html
42. CDC: Centers for Disease Control are different centers throughout the United States that are funded with private grant money from pharmaceutical companies to "discover fictitious disorders" and promote the pharmaceutical drugs.
43. *Families USA,* pp. 5,10
44. "Profiting from Pain where Prescription Drug Dollars Go" report by *Families USA*, July 2202, *New Scientist*, Washington
45. Follow the Money, The Pharmaceutical Industry – the other Drug Cartel, Office of the Minnesota Attorney general, Sept 30, 2003, p. 1
46. Kurt Langbein, p. 72
47. *New Scientist*, 17 Sept. 1994, p. 23 ff.
48. Langbein, p. 339
49. Cho, M.K., Bero, L.A., *The quality of Drug Studies, Published in Symposium Proceedings*, (Ann Intern Med 1996: 124 [5]), pp. 485-489

50. Robert S. Mendelsohn, *Confessions of a Medical Heretic*, (McGraw-Hill: 1980), p. 125
51. Der Spiegel 32/2005, p. 54
52. Der Spiegel, February, 2006, p. 156 f
53. Marcia Angell, M.D., *The Truth about the Drug Companies*, (New York: Random House, 2004), p. 198
54. Pharmaceutical Companies http://ushealthcarereform.com/page8.html Pulling Strings from Afar AARP Bulletin Today 2006-07-03 http://bulletin.aarp.org/yourworld/politics/articles/pulling_strings_from.html
55. http://www.saynotodrugs.org/
56. John Abramson, M.D., *Overdosed America, the Broken Promise of American Medicine,* HarperCollins Publishers, 2004, p. 90
57. Peter Weaver, *Smart Medicine, How to buy the prescription drugs you need a price you can afford*, (Nashville, TN: Rutledge Hill Press, 2004), p. 13

Chapter 3:

58. PDR https://www.pdrbookstore.com/Default.asp?
59. Formulary: the entire list of drugs available to the physician
60. Cornucopia: horn of plenty
61. United States Census Bureau, http://www.census.gov/prod/2001pubs/c2kbr01-10.pdf
62. Osteopathy: a system of medicine based on the theory that many diseases are caused by incorrect alignments of bones, ligaments, and muscles, and that correcting these through manipulation can cure the problems. It is often effective in treating joint and muscle disorders. MSN Encarta Online Dictionary
63. *MSN Encarta Online Dictionary.* http://encarta.msn.com/dictionary_/osteopathy.html
64. Lesley H. Curtis, Ph.D., Duke University Medical Center, Durham, N.C.
65. *Wall Street Journal,* May 21, 2004 for the year 2003.

66. TRENDS IN MANUFACTURER PRICES OF BRAND-NAME PRESCRIPTION DRUGS USED BY OLDER AMERICANS—2006 YEAR-END UPDATE – http://assets.aarp.org/rgcenter/health/dd154_drugprices.pdf
67. Taken from a chart prepared by the AARP Public Policy Institute and the *PRIME* Institute, University of Minnesota, based on data from Medi-Span Price-Chek PC (Indianapolis, IN: Wolters Kluwer Health Inc., February 2007). http://assets.aarp.org/rgcenter/health/dd154_drugprices.pdf
68. A *lipid* is a fatty substance in the blood. The lipid-lowering drug reduces cholesterol. A *platelet* is a component of blood. The *anti-platelet* drug prevents blood clots. *Osteoporosis* is a disease in which bones become brittle and likely to break. By keeping calcium out of the heart and blood vessel cells, the cells relax and chest pain and high blood pressure are controlled. A *gastrointestinal agent* controls stomach and bowel discomfort.
69. Source: AARP Public Policy Institute. TRENDS IN MANUFACTURER PRICES OF BRAND-NAME PRESCRIPTION DRUGS USED BY OLDER AMERICANS – 2006 YEAR-END UPDATE: http://assets.aarp.org/rgcenter/health/dd154_drugprices.pdf
70. While the vast majority of people in the program are the elderly, it also serves the disabled and, oddly, those with end-stage kidney disease. The latter was added because a USA lawmaker had a daughter with end-stage kidney disease.
71. *Medicare and Prescription Drug Costs-Part II*, http://www.therubins.com/medicare/drugcost2.htm
72. AARP: American Association of Retired Persons
73. AARP. http://Assets.aarp.org/rgcenter/post-import/2004_06_drugprices.pdf
74. AARP. http://Assets.aarp.org/rgcenter/post-import/dd112_brand_drugs.pdf
75. See footnote at 69

76. *Kathy Jones, "Drug Prices Increase Under Part D Plan" Families USA*, June 21, 2006
77. AARP, http://www.aarp.org/research/health/drugs/aresearch-import-656-DD77.html
78. http://www.aarp.org/research/health/drugs/aresearch-import-656-DD77.html
79. Source: information contained in the report "Enough to Make You Sick: Prescription Drug Prices for the Elderly" from *Families USA*
80. http://www.therubins.com/geninfo/eldpresc.htm
81. http://junkscience.com/news2/viagra4.htm
82. http://www.cnn.com/HEALTH/9805/22/viagra.patients/index.html
83. http://www.sddt.com/News/article.cfm?SourceCode=19980826fe
84. Christopher Gearon, "The Search for a Female Viagra," *Discovery*, http://health.discovery.com/centers/womens/viagra/viagra.html
85. Ibid.
86. ABC News, reported by BLTC, http://mdma.net/sexstasy
87. Karen S. Petersen, *USA Today,* March 21, 2001, http://www.usatoday.com/news/health/2001-03-21-viagra-abuse.htm
88. "Viagra May Cause Heart Attack Deaths In Younger Men With No heart Problems, Study Finds," *PSA Rising Magazine*, May 14, 2000, http://psa-rising.com/medicalpike/vaigracardiodeaths031500.htm
89. *Future*, http://www.globalchange.com/viagranews2.htm
90. Note: ADR increases exponentially with 4 or more medications. In the USA, 2.8 billion prescriptions were filled in the year 2000, which means about 10 prescriptions for every person in the United States. Adverse drug reactions kill over 100,000 plus Americans every year. Adverse drug reactions are already the No. 4 killer in the USA after heart disease, cancer and stroke.
91. Judith A. De Cava, *Cholesterol, Facts & Fantasies,* (Centerville, Massachusetts, 1994)

92. Lynne McTaggart, *What Doctors Don't Tell You*, (New York: Harper Collins, 2002)
93. Quotation found by Judith A. De Cava, p. 3
94. De Cava, p. 6
95. De Cava, p. 6
96. De Cava, p. 40, De Cava quoting Lynne Mc Taggart
97. Widgetal®: a made-up name for a drug. A "widget" is a mythical thing used for discussion in college business classes.
98. Pamela D. Larson and Janice L. Hoot Martin, "Polypharmacy and Elderly Patients," *AORN JOURNAL,* March 1999. Reported at http://www.findarticles.com/p/articles/mi_m0FSL/is_3_69/ai_54216921
99. Larson and Martin, Ibid.
100. Over-prescription of antibiotics has been blamed for the build up of drug resistant strains of bacteria. Ibid.
101. Larsen-Martin, Ibid.
102. R Stewart, W Hale, "Acute Confessional States in Older Adults and the Role of Polypharmacy," *Annual Review of Health* 13 (1992) p. 425
103. A Moraca-Sawicki, "Drug Therapy and the Older Adult," in *Pharmacotherapeutics: a Nursing Process Approach*, Ed M Kuhn (Philadelphia: F A Davis, 1998) p. 87
104. Larsen-Martin, Ibid.
105. Montamat, Cusack, "Overcoming Problems with Polypharmacy and Drug Misuse in the Elderly," *AORN Journal*, March 1999, p. 144
106. Infarct: an area of tissue that undergoes cell death due to lack of blood supply to the area
107. Der Spiegel 48/2005, p. 160
108. Josef Hasslberger, "Health Supreme," Reported at: http://www.newmediaexplorer.org/sepp/2004/01/31/lipitor_the_human_cost.htm
109. Drugs.Com http://www.drugs.com/cons/lipitor.html
110. Hasslberger, Ibid.
111. Drugs.Com, Ibid.
112. Larsen-Martin, Ibid.

113. Tracy McVeigh, "Tranquilizers 'More Lethal Than Heroin,'" *The Observer*, 5 Nov. 2000
114. Beverly K. Eakman, "Anything That Ails You, Women on Tranqs in a Self-Serve Society," *Chronicles*, Aug. 2004
115. "Some Psychotropics May Be Inappropriate for the Elderly," *Geriatric Times,* Vol. II, Issue 2, Mar./Apr. 2001; Mort JR, Aparasu RR, "Anti-anxiety Drugs and the Elderly; For Many, Psychiatric Medications Are Inappropriately Prescribed," *Archives of Internal Medicine,* Vol.106, 2000, pp. 2825-2831
116. "Elderly Abuse, Cruel Mental Health Programs," *Citizens Commission on Human Rights*, 2004
117. Ibid.
118. Ibid.
119. Akathisia is a movement disorder characterized by a feeling of inner restlessness and a compulsion to be in constant motion. Often a side effect of certain drugs.
120. Reported by Japanese researchers in *The Lancet*, the Journal of the British Medical Association, in 1998
121. Centenarians: people who are at least 100 years old

Kevin Snead Interview:

122. Note: In fact, John Abramson, who wrote *Overdosed America*, (HarperCollins Publishers, 2004) states "…for every 100 people with a history of cardiovascular disease treated with Vioxx instead of naproxen, there were between seven and 11 additional serious cardiovascular complications each year." Naproxen is a drug originally used to suppress the inflammation pain of arthritis.
123. Radical mastectomy: the removal of the breast, which has been diagnosed with cancer
124. Narconon: an organization that is highly successful in the rehabilitation of alcoholics and drug addicts
125. Reverse osmosis: a process used to purify the drinking water

Chapter 4:

126. Dr. Allan Greene, "A Welcome Revolution in Ear Infection Treatment," March 11, 2002 and http://www.drgreene.com/21_1771.html
127. Lyyne McTaggart, Ibid., p. 181
128. *Neomycin* is mainly used topically in the treatment of skin and mucous membrane infections, wounds, and burns. Although it is also used systemically, it is highly toxic. http://reference.allrefer.com/encyclopedia/N/neomycin.html
129. *Chloramphenicol* is used in the treatment of infections caused by bacteria. It works by killing bacteria or preventing their growth. http://health.yahoo.com/health/drug/202127/
130. Lynne McTaggart, p. 190
131. Lynne McTaggart, p. 191
132. Harris L. Coulter, *Vaccination, Social Violence, and Criminality,* (North Atlantic Books, California, 1990)
133. Sudden Infant Death Syndrome is also known as crib death. It is a fatal syndrome that affects sleeping infants under a year old, wherein the baby suddenly stops breathing.
134. Tim O'Shea, *The Sanctity of Human Blood, Vaccination is not Immunization,* (North Woods, 2003), p. 54
135. Lawrence K. Altman, "Smallpox Proposal Raises Ethical Issue," *The New York Times*, June 22, 2002
136. Andrew Wakefield and Associates, *The Lancet*, British Medical Journal, 1998
137. Rhinitis: inflammation of the mucous membrane of the nose
138. Coulter, p. 151
139. Coulter, p. 258
140. Mendelsohn, M.D., *How to Raise a Healthy Child In Spite Of Your Doctor,* (Ballantine, New York, 1984), p. 165
141. See Gary Null, ibid. p. 126

142. Tim O'Shea, *The Sanctity of Human Blood, Vaccination is not Immunization,* (North Woods, 2003), p. 62
143. See http://www.med-library.net/content/view/319/41/
144. Informed consent advocate says government and industry should release flue vaccine effectiveness data. http://www.vaccineinfo.net/immunization/vaccine/influenza/flu_vaccine_facts.shtml: "The flu vaccine only protects against the three specific viral strains which are included in any given year's flu vaccine. Throat, respiratory, gastrointestinal and ear infections caused by bacteria or other kinds of viruses are not prevented by getting an annual flu shot."
145. SSRI: (selective serotonin reuptake inhibitor) a class of drugs, such as fluoxetine or sertraline, that inhibit the uptake of serotonin by neurons of the central nervous system and are primarily used in the treatment of depression and obsessive compulsive disorder.
146. Minutes of the meeting convened by the Department of Health and Human Services Food and Drug Administration Center for Drug Evaluation and Research held on February 2, 2004, http://www.fda.gov/ohrms/dockets/ac/04/transcripts/4006T1.htm pp. 12 – 13.
147. http://www.fda.gov/ohrms/dockets/ac/04/transcripts/4006T1.htm p. 14
148. http://www.fda.gov/ohrms/dockets/ac/04/transcripts/4006T1.htm p. 21
149. In 2003, the USA New Freedom Commission on Mental Health recommended, as influenced by psychiatrists and psychologists, that there be "…early detection of mental health problems in children and adults – through routine and comprehensive testing and screening." – "Harming Youth, Psychiatry Destroys Young Minds," *CCHR*, 2004.
150. TODAY Show interview (27 June)
151. *PEOPLE Magazine*, (11 July)
152. http://www.chadd.org/fs/fsl.htm
153. Ibid.
154. Subluxations: a partial dislocation of a bone in a joint

155. *Ritalin* is a mild stimulant to the central nervous system (brain and nerves). The exact way that Ritalin works is unknown.
156. *Methylphenidate* is a mild stimulant to the central nervous system (brain and nerves). The exact way that methylphenidate works is unknown.
157. *Adderal* is a stimulant and appetite suppressant. It stimulates the central nervous system (nerves and brain) by increasing the amount of certain chemicals in the body. This increases heart rate and blood pressure and decreases appetite, among other effects.
158. Karen Hadley, "Singer Appeals to DCs for the Children," *The Chiropractic Journal*, August 2004
159. *The Communication Line*, 19 April 2005, p. 2.
160. Elyse Van Breemen, "Say NO To Mental Health Screening Of Teens," *The Communication Line*, 22 November 2005, pp. 1 – 2
161. http://hanseisenman.typepad.com/health/2006/02/suicidal_teens_.html#more
162. http://www.oneaddplace.com/famous.htm
163. "Harming Youth, Psychiatry Destroys Young Minds," *Citizens Commission on Human Rights*, 2004
164. *Vicodin* is indicated for the relief of moderate to moderately severe pain.
165. *OxyContin* is in a class of drugs called narcotic analgesics. It is a pain reliever.
166. See http://www.boston.com/yourlife/health/children/articles/2003/08/20/ most_drugs_never_tested_for_safety_in_children/
167. http://pubs.acs.org/subscribe/journals/mdd/v07/i03/pdf/304rules.pdf
168. *Prozac* is documented with having caused suicide in quite a few cases.
169. *Zoloft* is a drug used in the treatment of depression, panic disorder, obsessive-compulsive disorder, and post-traumatic stress disorder.

170. *Haldol* is an antipsychotic drug of high-potency, strong tranquilizer and is used in the treatment of acute psychosis, acute schizophrenia, manic phases, to control aggression, to control agitation, disorganized and psychotic thinking.
171. *Lithium* is an anti-manic agent used to treat manic-depression.

Dr. Benoit Choiniere Interview:

172. Cum laude: with honors
173. Electro-diagnosis: Electro-diagnostic studies include EMG and NCS. EMG uses inserted needles to trace the electrical activity of muscles and is used to diagnose nerve and muscle disorders. NCS, or nerve conduction studies, is a diagnostic tool that measures the rate at which an electrical impulse moves along a nerve. It is used to diagnose disorders of the peripheral nerves and muscle.
174. Biomechanical: the study of the mechanics of a living body, especially of the forces exerted by muscles and gravity on the skeletal structure
175. Contraindication: those things that make the taking of the drug inadvisable: for example an allergic reaction
176. Parkinson disease: a disorder of the nervous system that affects muscle control
177. Dopamine: the substance formed normally in the brain and essential to the normal function of the central nervous system. The reduction of this substance causes certain disease conditions.
178. Electrolytes: electrically charged particles in the body's cells that are necessary to maintain voltages across their cell membranes and to carry electrical impulses
179. Opiates: any of several sedative narcotics containing opium or one or more of its natural or synthetic derivatives

180. Amphetamines: a colorless, volatile liquid used as a central nervous system stimulant in the treatment of certain conditions
181. Methamphetamines are addictive stimulant drugs that strongly activate certain systems in the brain. They are closely related chemically to amphetamine but have greater central nervous system effects.

Chapter 5:

182. Dr. Thomas Röder, Volker Kubillus, *Die Männer hinter Hitler, (Men behind Hitler*), (Pi-Verlag: Malters, Switzerland: 1994), p. 45
183. R. von Krafft-Ebing, *Gerichtliche Psychopathologie*, (Stuttgart: 1982), p. 3
184. Röder, Kuillus, *Die Männer hinter Hitler (Men Behind Hitler),* (Malters, Seitzerland: Pi-Verlag: 1994), p. 52
185. Third Reich is Hitler's Regime, 1939 – 1945.
186. Röder, Kubillus, *The Men Behind Hitler*
187. *The Merck Manual*, Merck Research Laboratories: Rahway, N.J: 1992
188. http://www.prozac.com/disease_information/disease_information.jsp?reqNavId=1
189. NARSAD (National Alliance for Research on Schizophrenia and Depression) is a private, not-for-profit public charity organized for the purpose of raising funds for scientific research into the causes, cures, treatments and prevention of severe psychiatric brain disorders, such as schizophrenia and depression.
190. http://pubs.acs.org/subscribe/journals/mdd/v07/i03/pdf/304rules.pdf
191. Schmid LG, et al: Adverse drug reactions: an epidemiological study at psychiatric hospitals, *Acta Psychiatr Scand 70*, pp.77 – 89, 1984
192. Grasso, Rothschild, Genest, and Bates, *What Do We Know About Medication Errors in Inpatient Psychiatry,* Joint Commission Journal on Quality and Safety, 2003, p. 397

193. Idem.
194. Leape LL, et al: *The nature of adverse events in hospitalized patients: Results of the Harvard Medical Practice Study II*, N Engl. J Med 324, pp. 377 – 384, 1991
195. http://www.msnbc.msn.com/id/6254504
196. *S(elective) s(erotonin) r(euptake) i(nhibitor):* A class of drugs, such as fluoxetine or sertraline, that inhibit the uptake of serotonin by neurons of the central nervous system and are primarily used in the treatment of depression and obsessive compulsive disorder.
197. Akathisia manifests as pacing and a total inability to sit still. If forced to sit still the person experiences extreme anxiety and agitation. In bad cases the anxiety and agitation may get worse even while the person is moving. Akathisia is dangerous in that it couples an extremely unpleasant experience with an intense urge to act, possibly leading to suicide attempts.
198. Disinhibition: loss of inhibition, as through the influence of external stimuli such as drugs or alcohol, or as a result of brain damage
199. Lability: open to change; adaptable: *an emotionally labile person*
200. Depersonalization: in *Psychology,* a state in which the normal sense of personal identity and reality is lost
201. Peter R. Breggin, *Toxic Psychiatry*, (New York: St. Martins Press, 1991), p. 247
202. Third Reich: during 1933 to 1945, the German state under Adolf Hitler
203. Psycho-pharmaceuticals: drugs used in the treatment of emotional disorders
204. Filidei, "New Mental Health Initiative Forwards Psychiatry's Brave New World," *The Communication Line*, Clearwater, Florida: Creative Communications & Designs, Inc, 2004
205. Activated by or capable of liberating serotonin, especially in transmitting nerve impulses

206. Ann Blake Tracy, *Prozac: Panacea or Pandora?*, (Utah: Cassia Publications, 1994) http://members.aol.com/atracyphd/syndrome.htm
207. http://www.lef.org/fda/fdaban95.html
208. http://www.paxil-side-effects-lawsuits.com/pages/sideeffect.html
209. http://www.zoloft-suicide-side effects.com
210. http://www.wellbutrin-xl.com/benefits/wxl_low_sexual_side_effects.html

Dr. Whitaker Interview:

211. Statin drugs: Statin drugs are a class of drugs used to lower cholesterol levels in people who are at risk with cardiovascular disease.
212. Bipolar: A Psychiatrist-labeled disease in which a person feels the extremes of high and low emotion. The cause of this is unknown to the Psychiatric field.
213. Oxycontin: a prescription narcotic drug used to treat moderate to severe pain. It contains a controlled time-released formula to extend the pain relief over an extended amount of time.
214. Dilantin: a prescription drug commonly used for seizures.
215. GABA: a supplement that induces relaxation, analgesia and sleep. It is a substance that is normally manufactured in the brain.
216. Tryptophan: an essential amino acid that is not synthesized by humans, but is essential as part of our diet and is obtained from dietary proteins such as red meat, eggs, fish, poultry, milk, yogurt, and cottage cheese, as well as chocolate, oats, bananas, spirulina, peanuts, dried dates, mangoes, sesame, chickpeas, sunflower seeds, and pumpkin seeds. It is typically used as an effective sleep aid as well as an antidepressant.
217. Five hydroxyl-tryptophan: a naturally-occurring amino acid found in certain foods like turkey and cheese used

for depression and mood disorders as well as a sleep aid, antidepressant, and appetite suppressant.

218. Ritalin: a prescription stimulant drug commonly used to treat ADHD.
219. Zocor: a cholesterol-lowering medication
220. Zoloft: a medication used to treat depression, stress, anxiety and many other similar kinds of disorders.
221. Effexor: an antidepressant medication also used for anxiety, panic, etc..

Dr. Bolick Interview:

222. Radiology: the study of the use of x-rays as a diagnostic tool.
223. Attention Deficiency Disorder is a psychiatric invented mental illness to describe a condition in which a person is not able to focus attention, and who is depressed and emotionally unstable as well as disorganized due to some chemical imbalance in the brain. There is no scientific evidence that this condition actually exists.
224. Andropause: the condition in the male whereby there is a lowering of the testosterone in the body as they become elderly, something similar to what the female goes through at menopause
225. DSM: *Diagnostic and Statistical Manual of Mental Disorders*
226. ICD-9: *The International Classification of Diseases – ninth revision*. This book is compiled of diseases that medical doctors encounter in their practice.
227. DTs: delirium tremens, which is an acute episode of delirium caused by withdrawal or abstinence from alcohol following habitual excessive drinking
228. Detoxing: the process in which a body gets rid of toxins
229. Valerian root: a plant, which is used as a mild sedative to handle stress and anxiety and to aid sleep

Chapter 6:

230. Cutclip/Center, *Effective Public Relations*, (London: Prentice Hall, 1964), p. 253
231. http://www.aha.org/aha/content/2006/pdf/fastfacts2006.pdf
232. Agency for Healthcare Research and Quality
233. Source: Reuters, updated: July 28, 2004
234. Source: *http://www.alkalizeforhealth.net/Ldoctordeath.htm*
235. See http://md-jd.info/iom-011.htm and http://www.nypirg.org/patientsafety/medication.pdf
236. See updated study of Jennifer Warner, "Medical Errors Still Plague USA hospitals," http://women.webmd.com/news/20040727/medical-errors-plague-us-hospitals
237. In Germany alone, 52 thousand "medications" are on the market despite that WHO states that only 306 are really necessary.
238. http://www.heall.com/body/healthupdates/drugs/adversedrugs.html
239. Tom Clavin, "How you can protect yourself," May 23, 2004, http://www.parade.com/articles/editions/2004/edition_05-23-2004/featured_0
240. Dr, Joseph Mercola, "Serious and Fatal Drug reactions in USA Hospitals," http://articles.mercola.com/sites/articles/archive/2008/01/02/hospital-drug-reactions.aspx
241. *Amazing Medicines the Drug Companies Don't Want You to Discover*! (Tempe, Arizona: Medical Research Publishers, 1993,) p. 14
242. Ibid. p. 16.
243. Ibid. p. 18.

Dr. John Feulner Interview:

244. DPM: Doctor of Podiatric Medicine
245. Pronation: the turning or rotating of the foot so that the inner edge of the sole bears the body's weight

246. Pathology: the anatomy of functional manifestations of a disease
247. Plantar fasciitis: heel pain caused by various things such as inadequate flexibility in the calf muscles, lack of arch support, being overweight, suddenly increasing activity, and spending too much time on the feet
248. Bunion: a painful, inflamed swelling of the bursa (a sac or sac-like cavity containing lubricating fluid between the joint and tendon) at the first joint of the big toe, characterized by the enlargement of the joint and displacement of the toe
249. Hammertoes: toes, usually the second ones that are permanently flexed downward, resulting in a claw-like shape
250. Over-pronation: the turning or rotating of the foot so that the inner edge of the sole bears the body's weight – flat feet
251. Gait analysis: the study of how a person walks
252. Osteoarthritis: a form of arthritis, usually in older people, in which the cartilage in the joints is worn down
253. Heel spur: soft, bendable deposits of calcium that are the result of tension and inflammation in the heel
254. Neuroma: a tumor composed of nerve tissue creating an inflamed nerve
255. Shin splints: painful conditions of the shins caused by inflammation of the surrounding muscles
256. Rheumatoid arthritis: a chronic disease marked by stiffness and inflammation of the joints, weakness, loss of mobility, and deformity
257. Psoriasis: a noncontagious inflammatory skin disease characterized by recurring reddish patches covered with silvery scales
258. Motrin: a trademark name for *ibuprofen*
259. Feldene: a non-steroidal anti-inflammatory drug
260. Naprosyn: a non-steroidal anti-inflammatory drug used to relieve the inflammation, swelling, stiffness, and joint pain associated with rheumatoid arthritis, osteoarthritis and other pain related conditions

261. Ibuprofen: a commonly used non-steroidal anti-inflammatory drug used for inflammation and pain
262. Hepatic: acting on or occurring in the liver

Chapter 7:

263. Balco: Bay Area Laboratory Co-Operative that operates as a nutritional supplement lab. Balco allegedly provided baseball stars with illegal performance-enhancing drugs recently.
264. THG: a designer steroid *Tetrahydrogestrinone*, derived by some simple chemical modifications of two well known and athletically banned – synthetic steroids, called *trenbolone* and *gestinone,* http://www.usatoday.com/sports/olympics/athens/track/2004-07-17-jacobs-suspension_x.htm
265. "Athletics," *Sports Illustrated*, London, 04 August 1998
266. EPO: *erythropoietin*, a blood-boosting hormone that enhances stamina
267. *Hemopure* is the brand name for a blood substitute consisting of ultra purified, modified bovine hemoglobin suspended in a salt solution, which contains no red cells. It enhances tissues by increasing oxygen profusion
268. NFL: National Football League
269. NIDA: National Institute on Drug Abuse
270. *Creatine* is a natural substance found in the body that plays a powerful role in energy metabolism. Taking creatine gives you more energy and allows the taker to exercise longer with out tiring out.
271. NO2 is nitric oxide that triggers the body to an increased blood flow to the muscles. This normally occurs during exercise anyways but with NO2 this increased blood flow does not stop once exercise has ended. This gives the serious athlete the ability to build muscle around the clock if he so desired.
272. Der Spiegel 48/2005, p. 147

273. Sullivan/Song, "Are Drugs Winning The Games?" *Time Magazine,* 11 September 2000
274. http://www.southcoasttoday.com/daily/09-00/09-22-00/c01sp094.htm
275. http://www.sportsline.com/olympics/story/6786641
276. Alan Leshner, Ph.D., "Anabolic Steroid," *NIDA*, 2004 http://www.nida.nih.gov/PDF/RRSteroids.pdf
277. Linda Skidmore-Rath, *Mosby's Handbook of Herbs and Natural Supplements, 2nd Edition,* (St. Louis, Missouri: Mosby Inc, 2004,) pp. 325 – 326

Dr Greg Olson Interview:

278. Indigents: low-income people
279. NFL: National Football League
280. "The Juice is Loose," *Men's Fitness,* March 07, 2005
281. Dole: welfare
282. Liberal Arts: academic disciplines, such as languages, literature, history, philosophy, mathematics, and science, that provides information of general cultural concern
283. Chiropractic Neurology: the study of how nerves work and how chiropractic relates to the function of the nervous system
284. Dihydrotestosterone: an androgen (a steroid hormone that controls the development and maintenance of masculine characteristics) derived from testosterone and having tumor-suppressing capabilities useful in the treatment of certain breast cancers
285. Creatine is a substance naturally produced by the body that helps to improve muscle performance during exercise. It is naturally found in meat and fish but is also made by the liver, pancreas, and kidneys within the body itself.
286. Amino acids combine to form proteins and are necessary to build muscles.

287. Free radicals are atoms or group of atoms that has at least one unpaired electron and is therefore unstable and highly reactive. In animal tissues, free radicals can damage cells and are believed to accelerate the progression of cancer, cardiovascular disease and age-related diseases.
288. DNA: the basic material within the living cell that transmits the hereditary pattern
289. Anabolic steroids: a group of synthetic hormones developed from testosterone that promotes the storage of protein and the development of muscle tissue
290. Sally McNeal: one of the most popular and loved female bodybuilders who competed in wrestling
291. DEA: Drug Enforcement Administration

Chapter 8:

292. Tim O'Shea, p. 46
293. In the last Olympic Games (Athena), from 40 horses, four were found to have substances in their urine, not permitted by the rules, stimulating substances, hormone-like substances, see Olaf Stampf, Spiegel 46/2004, pf. 174

Chapter 9:

294. Michelle Meadows, "Why Drugs get pulled off the Market," http://www.fda.gov/fdac/2002/102-drug.html
295. Thromboembolism: the blocking of a blood vessel by a blood clot dislodged from its site of origin
296. http://www.healthcentral.com/ency/408/guides/000010.html
297. "FDA accused of silencing Vioxx warnings," see http://www.msnbc.msn.com/id/6205699
298. Uffe Ravnskov, "New cholesterol guidelines for converting healthy people into patients," http://www.ravnskov.nu/ncep_guidelines
299. Uffe Ravnskov, ibid. p. 4

300. http://www.bmj.com/cgi/content/full/325/7368/828
301. Idem.
302. Mike Adams, "Aspirin and painkiller drugs cause widespread stomach ulcer," http://www.newstarget.com/000202.html
303. http://uk.reuters.com/article/governmentfilingsnews/idUKN1928836020061219
304. Mike Adams, "Long term aspirin use leads to pancreatic cancer," Sept. 15, 2004, http://www.naturalnews.com/000688.html
305. Source: http://sciencedaily.com/releases/2004/01/040107074621.htm
306. http://www.nihtraining.com/ohsrsite/irb/attachments/5-10_serious_adverse_event_rep.htm
307. http://www.who.int/patientsafety/taxonomy/Report_Delphi_Survey_ICPS.pdf
308. http://drugtopics.modernmedicine.com/drugtopics/content/printContentPopup.jsp?id=121720
309. http://www.drugtopics.com/drugtopics/data/articlestandard//drugtopics/072007/405100/article.pdf
310. Stephen Cherniske, M.S., *Caffeine Blues,* (New York: Warner Books, 1998), p. 46
311. Stephen states in his book "caffeine is a biological poison used by plants as a pesticide." Eating the plant will cause damage to the central nervous system of the predator and can prove lethal. *Caffeine Blues,* (New York: Warner Books, 1998), pp 16 – 17.
312. Ibid. p. 15
313. Homocysteine is an amino acid used normally by the body in cellular metabolism and the manufacture of proteins. Elevated concentrations in the blood are thought to increase the risk for heart disease by damaging the lining of blood vessels and enhancing blood clotting.
314. Ibid. p. 20 R.N. Warren, "Metabolism of Xanthenes Alkaloids in Man," *Journal of Chronalography,* 1969; 40, pp. 468 – 69

315. Stephen Cherniske, *Caffeine Blues*, (New York: Warner Books, 1998), p. 54
316. Ibid. pp 97 – 98
317. Ibid. p. 120
318. Joe Graedon and Teresa Graedon, *Dangerous Drug Interactions*, (New York: St. Martins Paperbacks, 1999)
319. Ibid. p. 25
320. Marcia Angell, physician and former editor of the New England *Journal of Medicine*, now a senior lecturer in social medicine at Harvard University Medical School. See her book *The Truth about the Drug Companies: How They Deceive Us and What to Do about it*, (Random House) and see AARP Bulletin, Sept 2004, p. 18 and www.aarp.org/bulletin
321. Der Spiegel, 6/2005

Chapter 10:

322. For example, Joseph J. Sweere, *Golden Rules for Vibrant Health in Body, Mind, and Spirit*, (North Bergen, NJ: Basic Health Publications, 2004) or *Amazing Medicines, the Drug Companies Don't Want You to Discover*, (Tempe, Arizona: University Medical Research Publishers, 1993).
323. Linda Skidmore-Roth, *Mosby's Handbook of Herbs and Natural Supplements*, (St. Louis, Missouri: Mosby, 2001)
324. Udo Erasmus, *Fats that Heal, Fats that Kill*, (Burnaby, BC, Canada: Alive Books, 1993)
325. DebraLynn Dadd, *Home Safe Home*, (New York: Penguin Putman, 1997)
326. See Ray D. Strand, M.D., *What Your Doctor Doesn't Know About May be Killing You*, (Nashville, TN: Thomas Nelsen Publishers, 2002)
327. Robert S. Mendelsohn, *Confessions of a Medical Heretic*, (Chicago, Illinois: Contemporary Books, 1979)

328. C.W. Fetrow, Juan R. Avila, *Complementary and Alternative Medicines*, (Philadelphia: Lippencott Williams and Wilkins), reedited and brought up to date regularly
329. Ebola virus: an extremely contagious virus that causes an acute, highly fatal hemorrhagic fever. It is spread through contact with bodily fluids or secretions of infected persons and by airborne particles.
330. Nicolai Worm, *Daily Meat*, (Hamburg: Hamburg Press, 2002)
331. By "organic", we mean food and meat produced without antibiotics, hormones, chemical fertilizers and other such biotechnology. Such food must not be treated with sewage sludge or exposed to irradiation or mingled with genetically modified organisms.
332. Sally Fallon, *Nourishing Traditions*, (San Diego, CA: ProMotion Publishing, 1995), p 15
333. A glycemic index is found on the Internet at http://www.diabetesnet.com/diabetes_food_diet/glycemic_index.php
334. For a good explanation of vitamins see Judith A. DeCava, *The Real Truth About Vitamins and Antioxidants,* (Columbus, GA: Brentwood Christian Press, 1996).
335. *Amazing Medicines*, ibid. p 325

Dr. Shyler Neveaux Interview:

336. Tai chi: a Chinese system of meditative physical exercises used to improve and maintain good health, increase longevity and designed especially for self-defense and meditation
337. Qi gong: a Chinese system of combining breathing, mental focus, stretching, and movement to promote health, fitness, and relieve stress
338. A.P., D.O.M., A.I.T: Acupuncture Physician, Doctor of Oriental Medicine, Acupuncture Injection Therapist

339. Shiatsu: a form of therapeutic massage in which pressure is applied with the thumbs and palms to those areas of the body used in acupuncture
340. Homotoxicology: a approach that uses homeopathic remedies to rid the body of toxins that prevent its healing
341. Fibromyalgia: a syndrome characterized by chronic pain in the muscles and soft tissues surrounding joints, fatigue, and tenderness at specific sites in the body
342. Osteoporosis: a disease in which the bones become extremely porous, are subject to fracture, and heal slowly, occurring especially in women following menopause and often leading to curvature of the spine from vertebral collapse
343. Spinal stenosis is a narrowing or constriction of the passageway that the spinal cord goes through which results in pain.
344. Sciatica: pain along the sciatic nerve usually caused by a herniated disk of the lumbar (of, near, or situated in the part of the back and sides between the lowest ribs and the pelvis) region of the spine and radiating to the buttocks and to the back of the thigh
345. Lou Gerigs disease is a chronic, progressive disease marked by gradual degeneration of the nerve cells in the central nervous system that control voluntary muscle movement. The disorder causes muscle weakness and atrophy and usually results in death.
346. Raynauds syndrome: a condition resulting in discoloration of the fingers and/or the toes after exposure to changes in temperature (cold or hot) or emotional events
347. Scleroderma: a pathological thickening and hardening of the skin and internal organs
348. Homeostasis: the ability or tendency of an organism or cell to maintain internal equilibrium by adjusting its physiological processes
349. *Lipitor* is used to lower cholesterol and triglyceride (fat-like substances) levels in the blood.

350. *Piriformis syndrome* is a condition in which the piriformis muscle irritates the sciatic nerve, causing pain in the buttocks and referring pain along the course of the sciatic nerve. Pain is known as sciatica.
351. *Tendonitis*: the inflammation of the tendon
352. Cold laser: low energy lasers that penetrate deeply into the skin and work by improving metabolism, circulation and tissue healing
353. Cross fiber friction is massage that goes across the grain of the muscle in order to break down the adhesions between the parallel fibers within the muscle. This restores mobility and removes both toxins and deeply held patterns of tension.
354. *Ishial tuberosity*: The rough bony projection at the junction of the lower end of the body of the pelvic region
355. Heel spur is the more common name for plantar fascitiis. Plantar fasciitis refers to the inflammation of the plantar fascia (the tough, broad band of fibrous tissue located along the bottom surface of the foot that runs form the heel to the forefoot). Calcium deposits form when the plantar fascia pulls away from the heel area causing extreme pain.
356. *Bipolar Disorder*: A psychiatric disorder marked by alternating episodes of mania and depression
357. *Wobenzym* is a combination of purified, naturally occurring enzymes that have proven to help control joint inflammation, improve healthy circulation, enhance immune function, and speed the recovery from strains and sprains. Enzymes are substances within the body that enable vitamins, minerals or hormones to do their jobs.
358. Systemic: Relating to or affecting the entire body or an entire organism

Chapter 11:

359. Jordan S. Dubin, Joseph Brasco, *Restoring Your Digestive Health*, (New York, NY: Twin Streams, 2003), p 194

360. L. Ron Hubbard, *Clear body, Clear Mind*, (Los Angeles: Bridge Publications, 1990)
361. Dr. Sandra Dabot, *The Liver Cleansing Diet*, see www.liverdoctor.com

Gerd Schaller Interview:

Chapter 12:

362. National Vital Statistics Report for 2002, volume 53, Number 5, October 12, 2004 http://www.cdc.gov/nchs/data/nvsr/nvsr53/nvsr53_05acc.pdf
363. Cardiovascular means of, relating to, or involving the heart and the blood vessels
364. Sophie Petersen, Viv Peto and Mike Rayner, "Coronary Heart disease statistics," 2004 edition, British Heart Foundation Health Promotion Research Group, Department of Public Health, University of Oxford, http://www.heartstats.org/uploads/documents%5c2004pdf.pdf
365. *Your Heart: Questions you have... Answers you need*, (Allentown, PA: People's Medical Society, 1996) p. 69
366. Aspirin as a Therapeutic Agent in Cardiovascular Disease"; Charles H. Hennekens, MD; Mark L. Dyken, MD; ; Valentin Fuster, MD, American Heart Association, Inc. 1997, p. 1, "http://circ.ahajournals.org/cgi/content/full/96/8/2751#R18
367. http://www.medicinenet.com/drug_induced_liver_disease/page8.htm
368. http://www.newswise.com/p/articles/view/503846/ "The Harvard Health Letter" released Mar 2004
369. Angiogenesis means the formation of new blood vessels. Angiogenesis inhibitors are drugs that blocks angiogenesis in cancerous tissue, thus interfering with tumor growth or metastasis.
370. Angiogenesis Inhibitors in the Treatment of Cancer"; National Cancer Institute©; 2002 http://cis.nci.nih.gov/fact/7_42.htm

371. "Cancer Facts": National Cancer Institute©: 2004
372. "Cellular Medicine in Heart Disease," http://www.drrathresearch.org/lab_research/heart_disease.html
373. Raymond Kurzweil, *The 10% Solution for a Healthy Life*, (New York: Crown Publishers, Inc, 1993)
374. http://www.health-science-spirit.com/cancerdiversity.html
375. *Der Spiegel:* 41/2004 p. 160
376. Pygeum africanum: a tall evergreen tree from which tea is made from its bark to control urinary disorders in men
377. Suma: a South American herb used to help regulate and enhance your endocrine, nervous, digestive, cardiovascular and immune systems.
378. Paullinia cupana: an herb harvested from the Amazon rain forests, used to support mental alertness and fight fatigue.
379. Ginkgo biloba: derived from the leaves of the Ginkgo biloba tree, and used to treat blood flow disorders, mental decline (dementia), memory and concentration problems, asthma and allergies
380. Q10: a coenzyme useful as a heart disease remedy and as a treatment for a host of other ailments including cancer
381. Amazing Medicines, ibid. p. 104 and 135

Chapter 13:

382. Der Spiegel 39/2005
383. Der Spiegel 6/2005
384. Der Spiegel 8/2005
385. Der Spiegel 46/2004
386. Der Spiegel 7/2005

ADDRESSES OF THE INTERVIEWEES:

Dr. Ron Gilbert, DC
5949 17th Ave W.
Bradenton, FL 34209

Kenneth W. Thomas
125 N Lincoln Ave
Clearwater, FL 33755

Ulrich Sommer
30 Turner Street, # 806
Clearwater, FL 33756

Dr. Kevin Snead, DC
3638 Dickerson Pike
Nashville, TN 37207

Dr. Arlen Lieberman, DC
5689 Duluth Street
Golden Valley, MN 55422

Dr. Benoit Choiniere, DC
640 Industrial Pkwy.
Elkhart, IN 46514

Dr. Julian Whitaker, MD
Forward Nutrition
c/o Healthy Directions, LLC
P.O. Box 59750
Potomac, MD 20854

Dr. Channing C. Bolick, DC
The Bolick Wellness Clinic
500 E Horatio Avenue
Maitland, FL 32751

Dr. John Feulner, DPM
Florida Biomechanics Group
7730 Starkey Road
Largo, FL 33777

Dr. Greg Olson, DC
2305 Lowry Avenue North
Minneapolis, MN 55401

Dr. Shyler Neveaux, DOM
2401 West Bay Dr., Suite 116
Largo, FL 33770

Gerd Schaller / Nature Power
Göllheimer Str. 10
67308 Biedesheim
Germany

BIOGRAPHIES

Dr. Ron Gilbert, DC

Dr. Ron Gilbert is a full time Chiropractic Physician with twenty-four years of clinical experience, having treated over fifteen thousand patients. He is a Board Certified Chiropractic Sports Physician and Board eligible American Board Chiropractic Orthopedists.

As well as having been invited by internationally renowned Orthopedic and Neurosurgeons to observe numerous brain, cervical, and lumber spine surgeries, he has been the Chiropractor for numerous international celebrities, and also the Chiropractor for the Richmond Ballet.

He has held advisory positions with the Virginia State Supreme Court along with four major insurance companies. Dr. Gilbert is not only a former USPTA rated Tennis professional but has received awards from the Virginia Chiropractic Association (the Presidents Award) and the Pinellas County Chiropractic Society, as well as the Distinguished Service Award from the Central Virginia Chiropractic Society.

Dr. Gilbert has held many other positions and has served on many Boards including Central Virginia Chiropractic Society, Virginia Chiropractic Association, Pinellas County Chiropractic Society, America's Foundation for Chess: Tampa Bay Chapter, Virginia Kick Boxing Association, and YMCA Medical Advisory Committee.

Thousands of nutritional, rehabilitative and exercise programs have been designed and supervised by Dr. Gilbert with incredible life changing results for his patients.

His 24 years of practice has given him first-hand experience with a wide variety of conditions that have been largely contributed by drugs and their side effects. Having seen a large number of people masking a physical problem instead of handling the root of the difficulty, which never really fixes the body, he gave many lectures and wrote words of wisdom. This drove him to contribute to Side Effects so that he can help many more people make better choices in their health care and nutrition.

Kenneth W. Thomas, RN

As a full-time practicing Registered Nurse for 30 years, Ken Thomas has assessed and interviewed patients, treated wounds, dispensed medications, mixed intravenous solutions, applied ointments and lotions, and recorded their effectiveness on thousands of patients. 10 years ago he began to notice that many of the symptoms presented by patients were a direct result of medication side effects and soon found that a high rate of debilitating adverse effects and even death began to mount in number. His interest took him to research and observe just how much this was going in the national news and in medical journals. He began writing articles about the area of mental health and the proliferation of labeling people, namely children, with disorders versus diseases. Ken wrote articles on Physical illness vs. Mental Disorders, ADHD, Anxiety Disorder and Depression that were published on the internet. Ken has an RN license and practices in Florida. He also holds a Bachelor of Science in Marketing and Management, obtained while working 12 years for medical equipment manufacturers as a medical sales representative. In 2006 Ken also started an organization called Nurses for Human Rights to expose and discuss the issue of psychiatry's pharmaceutical assault on children. Ken works as an Expert Witness in the medical-legal field. Ken was born in 1955 in Clearwater, FL where he now resides and works, writes, and campaigns for human rights.

Articles he has written:

Teen Screen Calls Physical Illness a Mental Disorder – Sierra Times 2006

Is It Really ADHD? – La Leva di Archimede, 2006

Is It Really Anxiety Disorder? – Op Ed News, 2007

Gerd Schaller

Gerd Schaller, born in 1944, is known in many first-class companies as a top professional in direct marketing techniques. Some of his clients came from the upper tenth of the upper twentieth of economic prosperity.

Six years ago, one of his closest relatives became sick because of the side effects of pharmaceutical medications, and died. Because of that, Schaller started a completely new career, and devoted his life to the health industry. Today he is the Executive Director of a company that concentrates on nutritive supplements. His purpose is to help thousands and thousands of people retain their health – without the side effects of pharmaceutical products.

Schaller wrote extensively on health issues in books, articles, and widely-published newsletters – and gained opinion-leader status. He is also engaged in the *Research for Health Foundation* that gathers and publishes old and new natural therapies as well as nutritional therapies.

See: http:// research4health.com/

Or: http://www.naturheilkunde-lexikon.eu/1385.html